Essentials of Radiology

Essentials of Radiology

for

Medical Students and others
who find looking at radiographs
very difficult

P. M. BRETLAND
M.D., D.M.R.D., F.R.C.R.
Consultant Radiologist, Whittington Hospital, London
Honorary Senior Lecturer, University College Hospital Medical School, London

BUTTERWORTHS
LONDON AND BOSTON
Sydney — Wellington — Durban — Toronto

The Butterworth Group

United Kingdom	**Butterworth & Co (Publishers) Ltd**	
London	88 Kingsway, WC2B 6AB	
Australia	**Butterworths Pty Ltd**	
Sydney	586 Pacific Highway, Chatswood, NSW 2067	
	Also at Melbourne, Brisbane, Adelaide and Perth	
Canada	**Butterworth & Co (Canada) Ltd**	
Toronto	2265 Midland Avenue Scarborough, Ontario M1P 4S1	
New Zealand	**Butterworths of New Zealand Ltd**	
Wellington	T & W Young Building, 77–85 Customhouse Quay, 1 CPO Box 472	
South Africa	**Butterworth & Co (South Africa) (Pty) Ltd**	
Durban	152–154 Gale Street	
USA	**Butterworth (Publishers) Inc**	
Boston	19 Cummings Park, Woburn, Mass. 01801	

First published 1978

ISBN 0 407 00067 4

© Butterworth & Co (Publishers) Ltd 1978

British Library Cataloguing in Publication Data

Bretland, Peter Maynard
    Essentials of radiology.
    1. Radiology, Medical
    I. Title
    616.07'57   R895   77-30425

    ISBN 0-407-00067-4

Typeset by Butterworth Litho Preparation Department

Printed by J W Arrowsmith Ltd, Bristol

Contents

DEDICATION

To those undergraduate and postgraduate students whose audience reaction has governed the content of my teaching.

Preface

This book is based on the teaching of postgraduate and undergraduate students with which I have been engaged at the Whittington Hospital for the last few years. Clearly, it was impossible to teach the whole field of diagnostic radiology in the available sessions. I therefore offered a method of looking at x-ray films, one of systematic scrutiny based on anatomy, and illustrated by examples.

There are many books which offer first-class accounts of both general and specialized radiology, most of which are expensive, advanced, and chiefly for the radiologist — a few are written for the undergraduate or the junior postgraduate student. There is no intention to compete with any of these and, indeed, many are listed for further reading. What is offered in these pages is a different approach, as a start to making the best use of radiographic information.

In clinical teaching, the student is expected to learn to take a history and examine the patient, and to make certain simple investigations, but he is not required to perform sophisticated tests, nor to undertake difficult treatments. He will, however, be expected, after qualification, to sign x-ray request forms and to look at plain x-ray films, although special investigations will not normally reach him without a radiologist's report. For this reason, this book offers an elementary systematic method of looking at plain x-ray films, studying each group of structures in turn in order to establish the normal anatomy and take note of any deviation from normality. With the aid of such a system the plain film can be approached with some confidence that no significant sign will be missed.

It is also hoped that this anatomical and pathological approach will help the student in his three-dimensional understanding of what goes on inside his patient, and render certain concepts easier to visualize and understand.

It is thus for the student in his first clinical year that this book is written, but it may also prove of value to others who wish to improve their methods of examination, just as those preparing for higher qualifications in clinical branches of medicine are often advised to return to the study of elementary clinical methods as a starting point.

It must be emphasized that this book does not pretend to be a pocket textbook of radiology. Although it contains considerably more detail than other student texts, it does not offer complete coverage of the subject and there is in many places deliberate over-simplification in order to emphasize an important point of principle. The reader who has completed it should not be deceived into thinking that he has mastered the art of diagnostic radiology, but he will certainly have made a reasonable beginning.

I have been continually helped and encouraged by my senior colleague Dr. W. Stachurko, who has willingly continued to shoulder more than his share of the routine work of the department while I did the teaching, and who has read the manuscript and made many helpful suggestions. Dr. D. C. Bernstein has made neuroradiological observations which materially improved the chapter on the skull. I am grateful to Dr. P. D. B. Davies for his comments on the chapter on the chest from the point of view of a chest physician, to Mr. P. T. Savage for his surgical comments on the chapter dealing with the abdomen, to Mr. D. F. Paton for his orthopaedic comments on the bones' chapter and to Dr. W. R. Parkes for his guidance on the pneumoconioses and the loan of Figure 2.12.

I am indebted to those who taught me radiology — Colonel K. H. Harper, for so long Adviser to the British Army Medical Services in Radiology, and Dr. C. J. Hodson, then Director of Radiology at University College Hospital, London (now Professor of Radiology at Yale University), who was the first to teach the 'outline signs'.

The radiographic illustrations are nearly all taken from material seen in the course of routine practice in the past ten years at the Whittington Hospital, and therefore cannot be regarded as unusual examples. They also include a small number gained from personal experience in West Africa and the Far East and a few taken from the museum in the X-Ray Department here. They are selected in order to illustrate the scheme of scrutiny of the x-ray film and an occasional rarity has been included to make a point. The difficulties in reproducing x-ray films as photographic prints are well known to anyone who has ever been involved with such work, owing to the tremendous differences between the photographic properties of double-coated transparent x-ray films and the positive printing paper on which the blockmaker depends.

I am indebted to the photographic department of the Royal Society of Medicine for some of the prints, and to Mr. J. J. Smith of the Broadway Studios, Loughton, for others; but the bulk of the work has been undertaken by Mr. S. M. Boukhari of the Islington Health District Photographic Department at the Whittington Hospital and his assistants at different times — Mr. Huitson and Mr. C. J. Chandler. I am also most grateful for their continued efforts to achieve the optimum results in so many difficult photographic problems.

The patience and encouragement of my wife and family during the writing and associated activities cannot go without mention.

Finally, I must acknowledge the enormous help which the students, undergraduate and postgraduate, have given in their comments on the teaching they received, in assisting to model the content of the instruction.

My thanks are also due to the publishers for their co-operation in the preparation of this work.

P. M. Bretland

CHAPTER 1

Introduction

Diagnostic radiology is the study of the process of inferring from the scrutiny of an x-ray image on a film (radiograph) or on a fluoroscopic screen whether or not disease is present; and, if present what kind of disease. This process, though extremely valuable, is not simple, nor is it foolproof nor vastly more certain than some other diagnostic methods and it has its limitations, as will be seen; it also requires a considerable knowledge of anatomy and pathology. However, by following the relatively elementary steps suggested in the succeeding sections and chapters of this book, it should be possible to arrive at some reasonable conclusions after looking at an x-ray film. Experienced radiologists and clinicians often appear to work for a lot of the time using instant 'pattern recognition' but are always on their guard against the fallacies inherent in the practice of assuming that diseases have characteristic radiological appearances by which they can always be recognized. Those beginning the study of radiology should not attempt 'snap' or 'spot' diagnoses but apply systematic scrutiny and logic to the material they examine.

To be able to do this it is essential to understand how the radiographic image is produced and a brief note about x-rays, their production and properties and how they work in this respect is unfortunately necessary at this stage.

Production of x-rays

X-rays are electromagnetic radiations of the same kind as cosmic rays, gamma rays, ultraviolet rays, visible light, infrared rays, diathermy waves, microwaves, radar and radio waves. All these differ only in their photon energies. X-rays lie between gamma rays and ultraviolet rays and those in use in diagnostic work are usually within the range from 12,400 to 24,000 electron volts (eV). They are produced when a stream of electrons emitted from a heated cathode in an evacuated glass tube is accelerated by a high difference of potential (45–125 kV) towards the anode (*Figure 1.1*). Most of the energy in the electron beam is dissipated as heat and less than 1 per cent in the form of x-rays, produced when the electrons interact with the atoms in the anode. The heat produced is considerable and nowadays is usually dealt with by immersing the tube in oil of high specific heat. The x-rays spread out in all directions. Therefore, in order to control them the whole device is encased in a lead cylinder with a small window to which is attached a collimating device to limit the size of the beam at will. The lead casing absorbs the remainder of the x-rays. To prevent the anode overheating, it is usually made in the form of a flat wheel which rotates rapidly on an axis parallel to that of the tube so that only a small part receives the electron beam at any one time. It follows that the whole thing becomes relatively heavy and since it must be suspended in space so as to be aimed in virtually any direction in three dimensions some very heavy and expensive engineering is required. Numerous engineering and electronic refinements for different purposes are continually being developed.

Formation of the radiographic image

X-rays possess certain properties of which the most important for our purposes are that they travel in

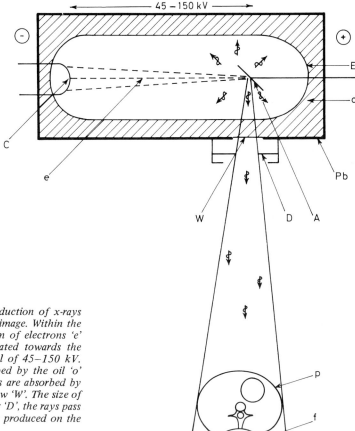

Figure 1.1   Diagram to show the production of x-rays and the formation of the radiographic image. Within the evacuated glass envelope 'E' the stream of electrons 'e' leaves the cathode 'C' and is accelerated towards the anode 'A' by a difference of potential of 45–150 kV. Heat generated in the anode is absorbed by the oil 'o' and x-rays ↝ emitted in all directions are absorbed by the lead casing 'Pb' except at the window 'W'. The size of the beam is controlled by the collimator 'D', the rays pass through the patient 'p' and an image is produced on the film 'f'.

straight lines and that they will pass through matter — but in differing amounts depending on the substance concerned and its physical state. All substances absorb or scatter x-rays to some extent (depending on the atomic number) and from this viewpoint it is possible to classify the tissues of the body into four main groups. The least amount of absorption is produced by *air* (or other gases), principally because they are gaseous and their atoms widely scattered. *Fat* absorbs rather more, but not as much as *water* and tissues which consist largely of water. This includes muscle, blood fluids of all kinds and solid organs such as liver, spleen and kidney. The greatest tissue absorber of x-rays is, of course, *bone*, principally on account of its calcium content but also because it is compact and solid. Finally, we may add heavy metals which may be on or in the person and the active constituents of contrast media (notably barium and iodine).

Only those x-rays which pass through the body reach the film. Those tissues which absorb or scatter a lot of x-rays are described as radiographically *dense*, and those which permit a lot to pass through are variously described as translucent, radiolucent or transradiant. *Transradiant* is the most logical term and will be used in this book.

The effect of x-rays on the conventional transparent x-ray film (as viewed on a white-light illuminator) is to blacken it. Consequently, we may make out a table of the four basic radiographic densities and their effect upon the film as shown in *Table 1.1*. Conventional x-ray film can easily distinguish these main groups but cannot normally show differences within them.

Examples of these different densities as seen on a normal chest x-ray film are illustrated in *Figure 1.2a* and *b*.

It thus becomes clear that the radiographic

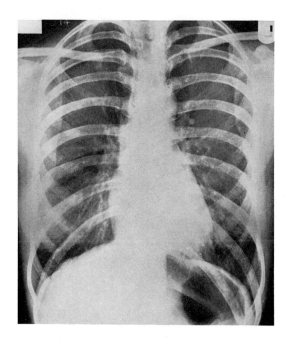

(a)

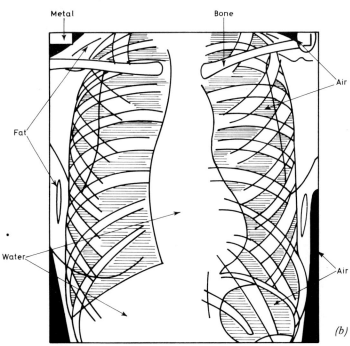

(b)

Figure 1.2   (a) Normal chest radiograph. (b) Diagram to illustrate the various radiographic densities seen on a normal chest film (a). Notice the air density outside the chest, in the lung fields and in the gastric air-bubble, and the fat between the muscle layers. There is no border visible between the shadows of water density of the heart and liver, but the ribs and spine are visible through the heart shadow. The most dense shadow is cast by the metal of the 'L' marker and that of the mask on the other corner which leaves a part of the film unexposed so that the name and date can be photographically printed on it.

Table 1.1

BASIC RADIOGRAPHIC DENSITIES

I Density group	II Tissue or location	III Effect on the film
(1) Air	Outside Body Air passages (mouth, throat, trachea and main bronchi) Lungs Gut (containing gas) and other hollow viscera Abnormal air spaces	Black
(2) Fat	Subcutaneous In deep fascia Around organs (for example, kidney) Apex of heart Medulla of bone Fatty tumours	Grey
(3) Water	Muscle Blood Heart shadow Liver, spleen, kidney and bladder Gut (full of fluid) Effusions Consolidations Ascites Cysts	Pale grey, often white
(4) Bone	Skeleton New bone formation Calcifications	Virtually white
Heavy metals and contrast media	Markers Metallic F.B.'s Organs demonstrated by barium or iodine compounds	White (no blackening — transparent film)

image is formed as a result of a pattern of differential absorption of x-rays and certain limitations are at once apparent — we cannot distinguish between gases, nor between blood or fluid in a pleural effusion, nor even between blood, heart muscle and pericardial effusion.

What has to be looked for and made use of is the radiographic contrast between the images cast on the film by the different types of tissue giving rise to visible borders or edges. It must also at once be apparent that the end result of many pathological processes will be to produce an appearance as of water density and that much will depend on the distribution and shape of the lesions; and the interpretation will depend on a knowledge of normal anatomy and of pathological processes.

CHAPTER 2 | # The Chest

INTRODUCTION

The chest is dealt with first because it is the commonest x-ray examination, because most doctors expect to look at a chest x-ray and understand it, because on account of its complex anatomy and diverse pathological appearances it can be amongst the most difficult to interpret correctly, and because some essential principles of radiological interpretation, of general application, can be introduced relatively painlessly. The intention in this chapter will not be to describe appearances in particular disease conditions but to help the student to establish the normal anatomy on the films he sees and to appreciate the changes from the normal in various structures. Descriptions of the radiological appearances in particular disease conditions should thus become relatively easy to understand and remember, based on knowledge of the pathological processes. The fact that some appearances are non-specific and are common to several diseases will become apparent.

RADIOGRAPHY

The most usual method of radiological examination is a plain PA film, so-called because the direction of the beam of x-rays is postero-anterior. The front of the patient's chest is applied to the film in its cassette and the x-ray tube is 5 or 6 feet (about 2 metres) behind him, centred on the 4th thoracic vertebra. The shoulders are pushed forward to displace the scapulae laterally so that they do not obscure the lung fields.

Before studying the film it is necessary to be sure that it has been taken correctly, in order not to be misled by unusual appearances due to the radiography but to recognize and take account of them. One must also be sure that it is the correct film of the correct patient. The following sequence of checks with practice will become automatic, done at a glance, or in a few seconds at most: (1) marking; (2) side; (3) position; (4) quality; and (5) respiration.

Marking

Look for the name of the patient — all films have to be marked with the name and date — and check that it is your patient and whether male or female. The nationality or race is worth noting as some diseases have geographical or racial associations, for example, hydatid disease in Cyprus, haemoglobinopathies in Greece and parts of Africa, tuberculosis in any developing country. Check the date and if there is more than one film, view each one in the right order.

Side

Look for the right or left marker, usually a single 'R' or 'L' seen on the appropriate side. In a PA film it is common for these to be reversed (or mirror imaged). Do not be misled by a dextrocardia.

Position

If the film is taken straight the medial ends of the clavicles should be equidistant from the mid-line, as also should be the anterior ends of the ribs. The line of the spinous processes may be deceptive; it is not always in the mid-line, for example, as in a patient with scoliosis.

Quality

If the radiographic factors have been correctly set by the radiographer it should be just possible to see the intervertebral disc spaces through the heart shadow. If the spine is seen too well, the film is 'overpenetrated' and the x-rays are 'too hard'; that is, of too high energy, generally due to a too high kilovoltage (kV) across the tube. If the film is too white and detail is generally poor, it is said to be 'too thin' or 'underpenetrated' and the x-rays 'too soft', generated by too low a kV across the tube; a somewhat similar appearance can be produced by underdeveloping.

Respiration

Although the duration of exposure is short (from 0.01 to 0.04 seconds on modern high power apparatus and even shorter on some special sets) the patient's breath must be held to avoid respiratory blur, though this may still occur with portable sets of lower power. Chest films are customarily taken during the deepest possible inspiration of which the patient is capable, for two reasons. First, this expands the lung as much as possible to reveal basal lesions which might otherwise be concealed and also reduces the size of the normal heart shadow to less than half the internal diameter of the thorax. Secondly, the position is reproducible on subsequent occasions in the same patient.

A deep inspiration should bring the right diaphragm below the anterior end of the 5th rib in the normal individual. Sometimes this is not possible — obesity, late pregnancy, ascites or other causes of distended abdomen, or decreased lung compliance may prevent it.

Now study *Plates 2.1* and *2.2* and decide whether or not the radiography is acceptable.

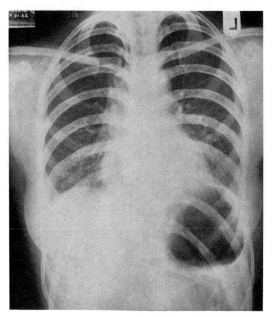

Plate 2.1

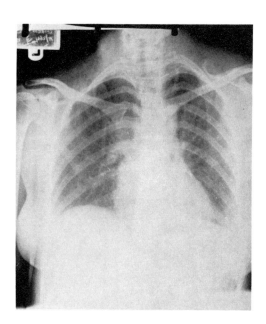

Plate 2.2

SOLUTIONS

Plate 2.1   Film taken in deep expiration. Note that only four anterior rib-ends are exposed above the diaphragm (same patient as in Figure 1.2a).

Plate 2.2   Dextrocardia (although the same effect could have been produced by incorrect side marking). Poor inspiration. Patient rotated, right shoulder forward.

Table 2.1

I Soft tissues	II Bony cage	III Central shadow	IV Hila	V Lung fields
(1) Root of neck	(1) Shoulder girdle	(1) Trachea	(1) Shape	(1) Pleura
(2) Axillae	(2) Vertebrae	(2) Super mediastinum	(2) Size	(2) Horizontal and other
(3) Pectoral muscles	(3) Ribs	(3) Heart shadow —	(3) Height	fissures
(4) Breasts	(4) Costal cartilages	size and shape	(4) Size of vessels	(3) Compare spaces
(5) Diaphragm and	(5) Sternum	(4) Behind heart	(5) Distribution of	(4) Peripheral lung
below		(5) Heart borders	vessels	pattern
				(5) Abnormal shadows

SCRUTINY OF THE CHEST FILM

The points to be looked at fall fairly conveniently into five groups of five, as summarized in *Table 2.1*.

SOFT TISSUES

Root of neck

The shadows of the muscles should be noted, also any swelling such as might be due to a goitre or abscess; calcifications may occur in tuberculous glands, thyroid adenomata or dead parasites such as guinea worms. Surgical emphysema can be seen and extraneous objects such as earrings or hair should be identified.

Axillae

Normally, only the anterior and posterior folds of the axillae are visible, but enlarged glands, inflammatory or neoplastic, may be seen — rarely, calcifications.

Pectoral muscles

Pectoral muscles are normally not obvious but if asymmetrical as in some manual workers there will be slightly more general density on (usually) the right side. Removal of all or part of the pectoralis major is done in radical mastectomy (rarely, even in the male) and this produces a relatively increased transradiancy on that side, that is, a darker lung field.

Breasts

Look carefully for the breast shadows in the female; the variability is so great that they can be missed. They should not be confused with the shadows produced by abdominal fat ('spare tyres'). An absent breast shadow may only be revealed by the greater transradiancy on that side; it usually indicates mastectomy for carcinoma, but unilateral gynaecomastia occurs in the male. Nipple shadows in either sex can be difficult. In the male they usually lie just beneath the 5th rib anteriorly (occasionally just above it) and in the female they can usually be located in relation to the breast shadow. If they are asymmetrical, there may be no alternative but to ask for a second film with small metal markers on the nipples to identify them.

Diaphragm and below

The right side of the diaphragm is normally about one rib space higher than the left; beneath it is the dense liver shadow. Beneath the left diaphragm is usually the gastric air-bubble medially, the spleen and the splenic flexure of the colon laterally, perhaps containing gas and faecal matter, but their relationship is somewhat variable. An absent gastric air-bubble usually indicates achalasia or hiatus hernia, provided the film has been taken in the erect posture. Either side of the diaphragm may be raised for several reasons: it may be paralysed. the liver may be enlarged, the splenic flexure may be distended, or there may be a lung infarct or a subphrenic abscess. A low flat diaphragm exposing the anterior ends of the 7th ribs is seen in emphysema but rarely can occur normally. Air under both sides of the diaphragm usually indicates perforation of a hollow viscus (though it may only be obvious on one side) but can also be seen after abdominal operations, penetrating wounds, pneumo-peritoneum or peritoneal dialysis. Small amounts of loculated gas can occur in subphrenic abscess and even in a liver abscess.* There are several varieties of diaphragmatic hernia, for example, traumatic hernia (usually through a central slit), hiatus hernia (through the oesophageal hiatus), Morgagni hernia (between the costal sternal attachments), and Bochdalek hernia (between the costal and vertebral attachments). The diaphragm is occasionally absent at birth (usually on the left).

There follows examples of abnormalities of the soft tissues (*Plates 2.3–2.10*). Allow yourself 15 seconds to look at each one and then compare your findings with the solutions.

* See also pages 65 and 66.

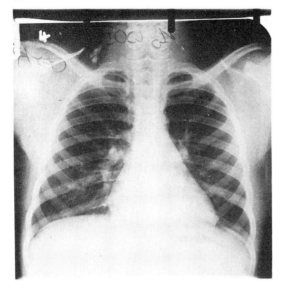

Plate 2.3

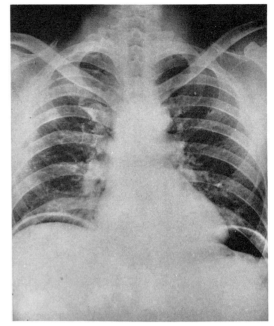

Plate 2.4

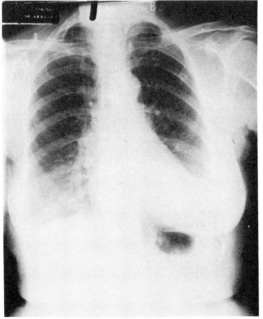

Plate 2.5

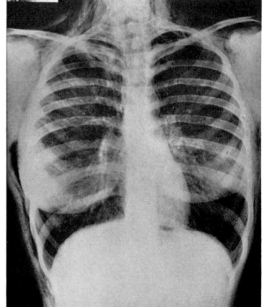

Plate 2.6

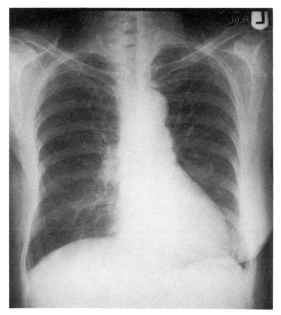

Plate 2.7

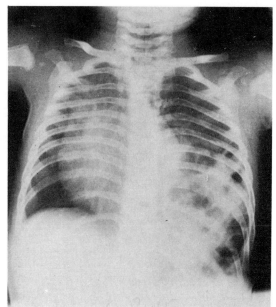

Plate 2.8

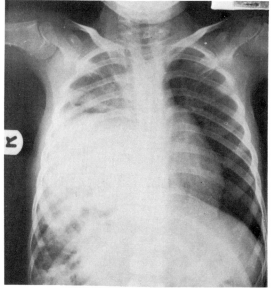

Plate 2.9

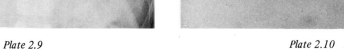

Plate 2.10

SOLUTIONS

Plate 2.3   Dense opacity in right side of root of neck. Old calcified guinea-worm (Dracunculus medinensis).

Plate 2.4   Gas beneath both diaphragms. Perforated peptic ulcer.

Plate 2.5   Irregular mass in left axilla. Increased density in medial part of left breast overlying heart shadow, which usually becomes less dense as it is traced laterally. Carcinoma of left breast with axillary metastases.

Plate 2.6   Transradiancies separating fascial and muscle layers in root of neck. Axillae and lateral to thoracic cage due to air; surgical emphysema. Thin layer of air alongside the left border of the mediastinum indicates a pneumomediastinum. This was a case of status asthmaticus. The increased intra-alveolar pressure caused air to track back along the peribronchial tissues into the mediastinum and thence out to the extrathoracic soft tissues.

Plate 2.7   Right breast shadow absent following right mastectomy for carcinoma.

Plate 2.8   Absent left hemidiaphragm in a neonate, with herniation of gut into thoracic cavity on the left and displacement of the heart to the right — acquired dextrocardia.

Plate 2.9   Right diaphragmatic outline difficult to see but at first sight looks raised; in fact, liver is in right hemithorax due to traumatic diaphragmatic hernia, confirmed by lateral view (Plate 2.11).

Plate 2.10   Right diaphragmatic outline appears raised; cause is not obvious in PA view. In lateral view there is a mass anteriorly and the barium follow-through (Plate 2.12) shows that it contains colon. This is a Morgagni hernia.

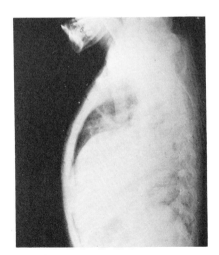

Plate 2.11

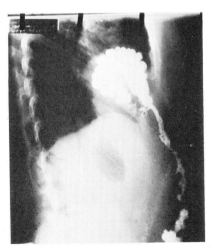

Plate 2.12

BONY CAGE

Bone involvement in disease may be local or general. It is therefore important to look both for individual bone lesions, and for generalized bone conditions such as congenital bone disease, metabolic bone disease or generalized neoplastic involvement as in metastatic disease from secondary carcinoma or myelomatosis. Malignant disease may be manifested by localized or generalized bony rarefaction or sclerosis (if neoplasm is suspected, it is essential to consider whether it is benign or malignant, and if malignant whether it is primary or secondary). Systematic scrutiny is clearly essential to avoid missing any detail, but this should not take long after some practice.

Shoulder girdle

The shoulder girdle includes the scapulae, the clavicles and the upper ends of the humeri where visible. The scapulae should be displaced laterally but this is not always achieved and the vertebral borders of the scapulae often produce lines down the lateral part of the chest which can be confusing unless already looked for and identified. The inferior angles are usually easily visible and occasionally contain transradiancies due to metastases; chondroma occurs in congenital bone disease (diaphyseal aclasia); Looser's zones (pseudofractures) can be seen in the axillary border in osteomalacia. The clavicles show bilateral medial defects in the congenital condition cleidocranial dysostosis, they commonly fracture and are occasionally the site of metastases or infection, for example, tuberculosis of the sterno-clavicular joint. The upper ends of the humeri are frequently abnormal in the elderly. Osteoarthritis, rheumatoid arthritis or old fractures or dislocations may produce quite bizarre appearances. Paget's disease, with its thickened dense cortex, may be seen.

Vertebrae

The lower cervical and thoracic vertebrae should be viewed rapidly from above downwards, noting any general alteration in alignment such as the smooth curve of a congenital scoliosis, or the angle sometimes seen in lateral wedging of a vertebral body as in tuberculous or other inflammatory disease, or collapse from injury, neoplasm or other cause, or even a congenital herni-vertebra. Neoplasm may also cause bony defects. Paravertebral masses may be partly visible though they are often concealed by the central shadow. Osteoarthritic changes with disc-space narrowing and osteophytic 'lipping' (common in old age) are usually noticeable, and it is always worth looking at the transverse processes as they may otherwise be mistaken for lung lesions.* The transverse processes of C7 point downwards, which allows it to be distinguished from T1 (the transverse processes of which point upwards); the presence or absence of cervical rib should also be noted.

Ribs

First, have a general look at the shape of the rib cage. The expanded rib cage in patients with emphysema or severe asthma, particularly involving the upper zones, may look almost square or oblong. A tall, slender, tapering, upper zone is generally seen in Marfan's syndrome but it can also appear in the normal. The bell-shaped chest in severe osteomalacia due to numerous pseudofractures of the lower ribs should be recognized, and a steep downward slope of straight anterior ribs may suggest a depressed sternum. In a severe kyphosis the upper ribs are superimposed.

It is best then to examine the rib appearances in three ways — first the posterior parts, then the anterior parts and, finally, the lateral chest wall (often seen better by holding the film with the spine horizontal), first one side, then the other. General changes in bone density or trabeculation should be observed and distinguished from overlying lung markings. The normal, often wavy, inferior flanges of the middle ribs should not be mistaken for pathology but notches in the lower borders of the ribs, classically associated with coarctation of the aorta and due to enlarged tortuous intercostal arteries as part of the collateral circulation to bypass the obstruction, should be specifically looked for. They do not occur in the upper two ribs — an observation entirely predictable from the origin of the upper two intercostal arteries from the subclavian artery. There are other, rarer, causes of rib notching (for example, in neurofibromatosis, arteriosclerosis involving intercostal arteries, obstruction of the inferior vena cava and after certain cardiac operations). Fractures, old or recent, traumatic (particularly in babies when they may be due to non-accidental injury) or pathological, bony defects from infection or neoplasm and periosteal reactions

*In ankylosing spondylitis the typical 'bamboo spine' may be seen and the costo-vertebral articulations may be fused.

from infection, or Caffey's disease in infants, may also be seen.* The characteristic, irregular, string-like appearance of a regenerated rib after sub-periosteal resection at thoracotomy should be readily recognized. There are also several types of congenital variation of ribs of no clinical signi-ficance, for example, spatulate or bifid anterior ends, or fusion of two ribs posteriorly. More gross abnormalities are usually associated with spinal deformities, and asymmetry of rib spaces may be the first sign of such conditions.

Costal cartilages

It is worth taking a deliberate look at the costal cartilages. In many cases they are invisible but the first is usually calcified in a pattern highly specific for the individual. Indeed, the shape and appear-ances of C7, T1 and the 1st ribs with their costal cartilages are almost as specific as a fingerprint in the identification of a chest film when there is any query about correct marking. Calcification of other costal cartilages has to be distinguished from other calcifications in the chest, usually by position

*Rib destruction associated with a mass in the lung apex is an essential part of Pancoast's syndrome (upper lobe neoplasm with shoulder pain, Horner's syndrome and wasting of the small muscles of the hand due to nerve involvement).

and general direction of the lines, but occasionally it takes bizarre forms and shapes and may need views in other directions (for example, lateral and oblique films, even fluoroscopy) to be sure.

Sternum

Usually the sternum is invisible in a straight plain PA film but slight rotation will bring the lateral margin of the manubrium into view; it can, as a rule, be identified by its shape and its relation to the medial end of the clavicle and should not be mistaken for an upper mediastinal tumour. Rarely, neoplastic erosions occur; fractures are usually seen only in the lateral view. In the infant, the sternum is represented by a row of rounded ossific centres, rather like a toy soldier's large tunic buttons, and can be particularly confusing if some rotation is present. If they have been thought about and carefully identified, no confusion need exist.

Plates 2.13–2.20 show some bony lesions, which should be fairly easily identified in a 15-second scan, bearing in mind the foregoing notes; but the reader is advised to look at the radiography and soft tissues first because in some cases it may be possible to 'put two and two together' and from the available evidence suggest a definitive diagnosis rather than a list of differential diagnoses which is all that is possible in others.

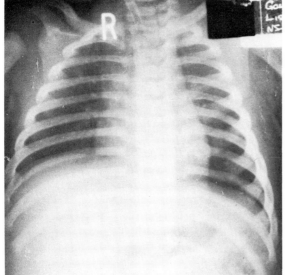

Plate 2.13

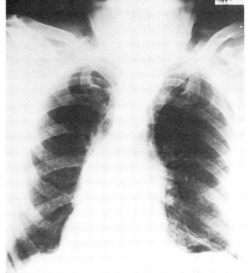

Plate 2.14

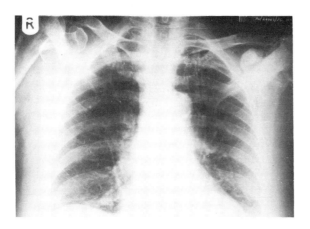

Plate 2.15

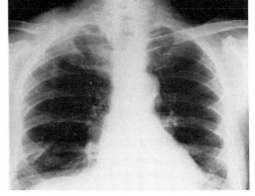

Plate 2.16

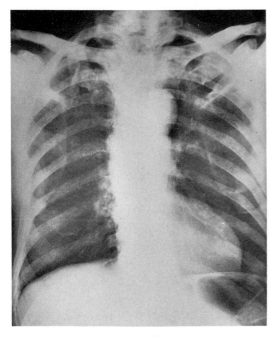

Plate 2.17

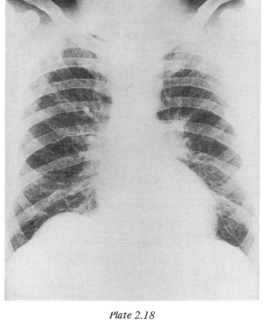
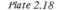

Plate 2.18

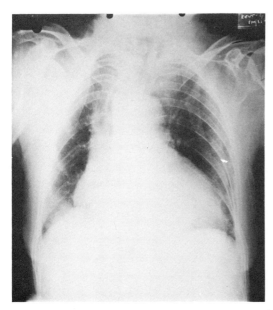

Plate 2.19

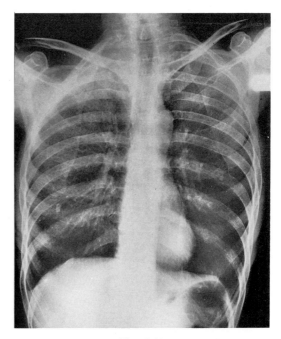

Plate 2.20

SOLUTIONS

Plate 2.13   Fusiform enlargements of the 6th, 7th and 8th ribs near their posterior ends; healing rib fractures due to non-accidental injury – 'battered baby'.

Plate 2.14   Thoracic scoliosis concave to left. Although the spine is largely concealed by the mediastinum, its convexity to the right is just visible and the medial ends of the left posterior ribs can be seen through the upper part of the heart shadow.

Plate 2.15   Subacromial dislocation of the right shoulder. Note also poor inspiration and rotation of right shoulder forward; this exaggerates the heart size but there is some increase due to left ventricular enlargement.

Plate 2.16   Defective medial half of right clavicle associated with soft-tissue mass. Edges of remaining part of clavicle are ill-defined with some loss of cortex and probable periosteal elevation inferiorly. It looks neoplastic and was due to a secondary deposit from carcinoma of bladder.

Plate 2.17   Generalized increased density, irregular in places, of all the bones; mixed sclerotic and lytic secondary deposits. Much better seen in other bones (for example, the pelvis, Plate 2.21) but the chest film should raise a suspicion.

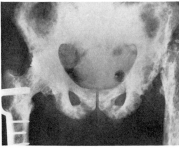

Plate 2.21

Plate 2.18   Notching of the inferior surfaces of several ribs associated with a large left ventricle which indicates coarctation of the aorta.

Plate 2.19   Abnormal left shoulder with thickening of cortex of acromion process, spine and coracoid process of scapula. Typical appearance of Paget's disease.

Plate 2.20   Soft-tissue shadowing in the right apex, with destruction of the posterior part of the right 3rd rib and associated transverse process, and part of the 2nd rib. Classical appearance of Pancoast's syndrome – carcinoma of lung apex with bone destruction, pain, Horner's syndrome and atrophy of the small muscles of the hand.

THE CENTRAL SHADOW

Some of the features to be looked for under this heading may have been noted *en passant* when surveying the root of the neck and the vertebrae; a second look now will enable them to be more accurately placed and/or the possibilities more extensively considered.

Trachea

The normal trachea should be seen as a vertical transradiancy, a dark shadow superimposed on the bodies of the cervical vertebrae. Its upper end is often seen, usually over the body of C4 (though this is somewhat variable, depending not only on the individual but also on the angle of the cervical spine to the vertical at the time of radiography) and has a curved arched appearance (Norman arch). It can certainly be followed down to the suprasternal notch and in a well penetrated film as far as the carina. Alteration in the upper end may be seen in laryngeal tumours (especially in the subglottic region) and displacements and narrowings occur in the presence of neck tumours, notably tumours of the thyroid, of which the soft tissue shadow may be visible. Mediastinal displacements (whether from pleural effusion, tension pneumothorax or obstructive emphysema ('pushing') or lung fibrosis or collapse ('pulling') may by shift of the carina displace it to one side or the other. Upper lobe fibrosis and shrinkage pulls the trachea into a curve convex to the affected side, while the other conditions are more likely to shift the carina and thus incline the trachea which remains relatively straight. The trachea is normally displaced slightly to the right by the aortic arch, more so if the aorta is markedly tortuous and arteriosclerotic as in the elderly. Asymmetrical masses in the mediastinum will also displace the trachea, as will an aneurysm of the aortic arch.

The superior mediastinum

The secret of making sense of this region is to consider the normal structures in it, determine how pathology could affect the appearances of such structures and decide finally what abnormal masses could occur. The normal anatomy, from before backwards, consists of retrosternal fat and lymph glands and the internal mammary (internal thoracic) artery, the thymus or its remnants, the superior vena cava on the right (behind the right border of the sternum and the first costal cartilage and thus normally providing the right border) with the right and left innominate (brachiocephalic) veins draining into it from above, still behind the manubrium. The ascending aorta and its main branches lie more medially, the aortic arch passing backwards and normally projecting a little to the left to form the so-called 'aortic knuckle'. The trachea passes downwards to the right of the aortic arch with the oesophagus behind it, the phrenic and vagus nerves descending on the lateral aspects of the main structures but in front of the hila. Posteriorly lie the descending aorta (lying initially to the left but lower down passing behind and to the right of the normal oesophagus), the prevertebral fascia, the spine itself and the sympathetic chain on each side.

It is often helpful to think of the mediastinum in three parts; an anterior part, in which a cyst or tumour of the thymus may occur, enlarged lymph glands, dermoid tumour or retrosternal goitre; a middle part in which aortic or innominate aneurysm, enlarged superior vena cava or dilatation of the oesophagus may be seen, and a posterior part in which neural tumours such as neurofibroma or ganglioneuroma, or paravertebral masses due to tuberculous abscess, eosinophilic granuloma or other spinal lesion may be the cause. Lymph gland enlargements may be inflammatory or neoplastic and may appear anywhere in the mediastinum.

There are certain features which, if present, can be helpful in identification. A small single lump of calcification is common in thyroid adenoma and thus may be seen in a retrosternal goitre. The aortic knuckle is often calcified in its left border in arteriosclerosis — very common indeed in the elderly. Lymph glands when enlarged in a group often have a lobulated outline. The dilated oesophagus, as in achalasia of the cardia, casts a curved shadow to the right; it often contains food residues which have a characteristic speckled appearance and a fluid level above which can be seen an air shadow and thick walls. Tumours of neural origin are frequently associated with pressure erosion of bone, in ribs or spine, but this may also occur with aneurysms of the descending aorta. The latter often have a lateral rim of calcification. Dermoid cysts may contain teeth. The thymus is often wider than the heart shadow at birth and may remain enlarged up to the age of 1 year, though it is rare for it to persist for long after this. If it projects more to the right, it often has a sail-like shape, resembling the back of a mainsail; on the left the outline is usually more rounded. This is a normal appearance, but if it fails to disappear between the ages of 1 and 2 years, further investigation is indicated.

The heart shadow

In the assessment of heart disease the appearance of the heart shadow on the PA chest radiograph is best studied in detail in relation to cardiology as a whole and only very basic observations are mentioned here. Two things should be noted, the size and the shape.

The heart size

Provided there has been a deep inspiration, the transverse diameter of the heart should not exceed half the widest internal diameter of the thorax, measured from the insides of the rib cage just above the costophrenic angle (in the infant, the figure for this cardiothoracic ratio is 0.64, reducing to 0.5 by the end of the second year). Any heart larger than this should be regarded as abnormal; however, a heart can still be abnormal with a cardiothoracic ratio less than 0.5; this may be seen in the narrow hearts associated with peripheral lung disease, particularly where the rib cage is expanded and the diaphragm low, and also in cases where enlargement has occurred in a relatively small heart but the transverse diameter has not yet reached half that of the thorax.

THE HEART SHAPE

The heart borders are normally composed of the various chambers, as shown in *Figure 2.1,* and selective enlargement of these tends to produce certain characteristic shapes.

The right heart border   This normally consists of ascending aorta and right atrium. If the aorta projects more to the right, then an aneurysm is possible but a similar appearance can be produced by a tortuous or unfolded aorta. Calcification of the right border of the ascending aorta is almost always associated with syphilitic aortitis. A projection of the lower part, particularly if there is a double shadow, is more likely to be due to enlargement of the left atrium projecting upwards and outwards behind the right atrium, although right atrial enlargement may also be seen on this border.

The left heart border   This is formed, from above downwards, by the aortic knuckle, the pulmonary conus (variously also known as the pulmonary segment or pulmonary bay and, depending on the type of heart, corresponding to either the outflow tract of the right ventricle or the origin of the pulmonary artery), the auricular appendage of the left atrium, and the left ventricle. The anterior border of the interventricular septum lies medial

to the left border in the normal heart, so that the right ventricle does not form part of either border.

It follows that a small or large aortic knuckle or a prominence of the pulmonary conus or left atrium (whose outlines are normally concave) can be fairly easily identified. An enlarged left ventricle, however, tends to enlarge generally downwards and to the left, whereas an enlarged right ventricle seems to produce a rotatory effect and the left heart border appears to enlarge upwards and to the left. Certain combinations of these prominences make some classical heart shapes, as shown in *Figure 2.2.* A small aortic knuckle and a large left atrium (LA+) indicate mitral stenosis, but if the left ventricle is also

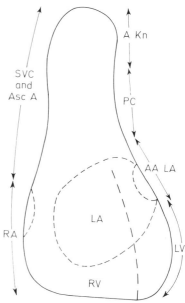

Figure 2.1   Diagram to show the parts of the heart borders on a PA view of the chest which correspond to the chambers and main vessels.

RA *Right atrium*	*PC* *Pulmonary conus,*
Asc A *Ascending aorta*	*segment or bay*
SVC *Superior vena cava*	*AA* *Auricular appendage*
A Kn *Aortic knuckle or*	*LA* *Left atrium*
knob	*RV* *Right ventricle*
	LV *Left ventricle*

enlarged (LV+) it would also suggest mitral incompetence. Enlargement of pulmonary conus is commonly seen with right ventricular enlargement (RV+), as in congenital heart disease with left to right shunt or in peripheral lung disease, although a prominent pulmonary conus alone can occur normally in young women, especially when pregnant, and also in thyrotoxicosis. Pure LV+ is commonly seen in hypertension, coarctation of

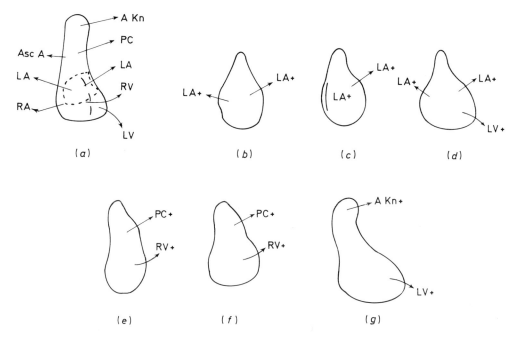

Figure 2.2   (a) Diagram to show the directions in which chambers of the heart and great vessels tend to expand on enlargement. Key as in Figure 2.1. Some basic heart shapes are shown in Figures 2.22 to 2.25 (b) to (e). (b) Mitral stenosis: LA prominent on both borders. (c) LA prominent on left border but only shown on right border by dense shadow inside border. (d) Mitral stenosis and incompetence: LA prominent on both borders but LV enlarged also. (e) Right ventricular enlargement; heart narrow, common in peripheral lung disease. (f) Transverse diameter increased, common in left to right shunts. (g) Left ventricular enlargement: transverse diameter increased.

the aorta, and aortic valvular stenosis and/or regurgitation; if associated with mural calcification of the ascending aorta it would suggest syphilitic aortitis with regurgitation.

There are other combinations which belong to the spheres of specialized cardiology, but the shape of the heart is sometimes unhelpful and angiocardiography may eventually be needed. Non-specific enlargement occurs in heart failure, cardiomyopathy or pericardial effusion, since the radiographic density of pericardial fluid is the same as that of blood and muscle.

CALCIFICATION

Calcifications within the heart shadow may be due to calcified mitral or aortic valves or the mitral valve ring, but can also be due to old calcified lymph glands behind the heart. Calcifications near the periphery may be in coronary arteries but if extensive, with an unusual heart shape, may be due to constrictive pericarditis. Calcification may also be seen in old myocardial infarcts, especially if they give rise to a localized aneurysm.

Shadows behind the heart

As mentioned previously, it should be just possible to see the thoracic spine through the heart shadow, certainly its left border; the ribs and the descending branches of the left pulmonary artery should also be just visible. A deliberate attempt should be made to identify these normal structures and to look for pathology. A tortuous arteriosclerotic aorta is often identified by a rim of calcification, a hiatus hernia by its air–fluid level and a collapsed left lower lobe by the disappearance of the left border of the spine with a dense triangular shadow against it. Tumour masses in the lung or neural tumours may also be seen.

Plates 2.22–2.32 are concerned with the central shadow and will require some thought.

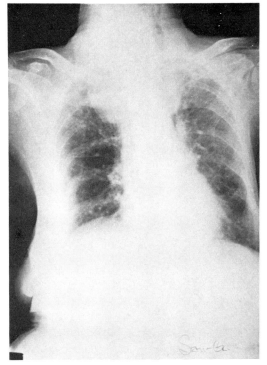

Plate 2.22

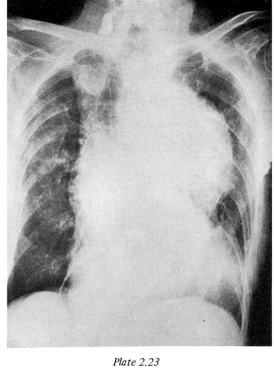
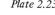

Plate 2.23

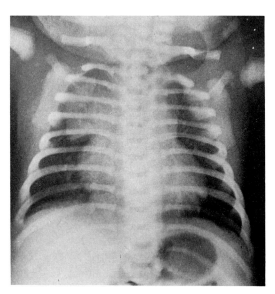

Plate 2.24

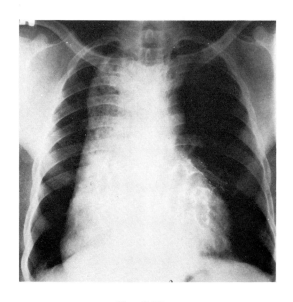

Plate 2.25

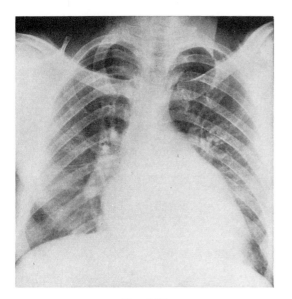

Plate 2.26

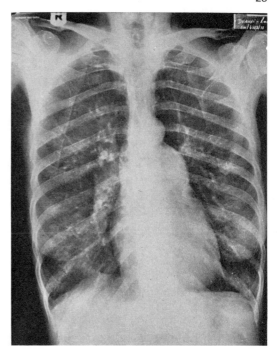

Plate 2.27

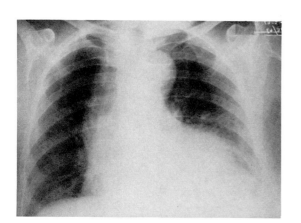

Plate 2.28

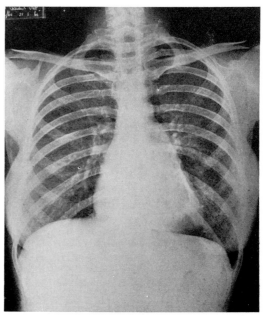

Plate 2.29

SOLUTIONS

Plate 2.22   Trachea is displaced and bowed convex to the left. There are soft-tissue masses on both sides of the neck (much larger on the right) continuing downwards. An enlarged thyroid with retrosternal extension is the cause. There is also slight left ventricular enlargement.

Plate 2.23   Massive aneurysm of the aortic arch and descending aorta, with some involvement of the ascending aorta. Note calcification of the ascending aorta − suggesting syphilis − and of the remainder of the aneurysmal wall. The trachea is displaced to the right; the normal aortic knuckle cannot be seen. The heart is enlarged due to left ventricular enlargement, presumably due to aortic incompetence; a calcification in the root of the neck is probably in a lymph gland.

Plate 2.24   Large thymus in a baby − normal appearance. A round transradiancy over the left clavicle is due to an entry port in the plastic roof of the incubator.

Plate 2.26   The heart is enlarged with prominences on the right and left heart border corresponding to the positions of the left atrium and its auricular appendage respectively; the aortic knuckle is small. Typical heart shape of mitral stenosis. Film slightly rotated, right shoulder forwards.

Plate 2.27   The transverse diameter of the heart is at the upper limit of normal, and there is considerable prominence of the pulmonary conus − typical appearance of right ventricular enlargement. In this case it is associated with peripheral lung disease, probably with some generalized emphysema; poor peripheral lung markings with low flat diaphragms.

Plate 2.28   Dense shadow behind the heart; it looks continuous with the descending aorta and might therefore be an aneurysm or a tortuous arteriosclerotic aorta; other rounded masses are also possible. It is just possible to make out an ill-defined right border to the shadow which means it must be in front of the spine. An over-penetrated film shows that it contains a fluid level and is in fact, a hiatus hernia (see Plate 2.31).

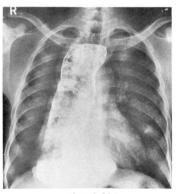
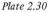

Plate 2.30

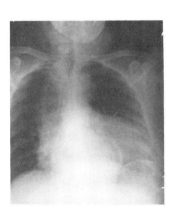

Plate 2.31

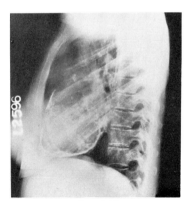

Plate 2.32

Plate 2.25   Mediastinal shadow is widened to the right all the way down and shows a curiously speckled appearance in its right part. It is just possible to see air shadows on each side of the trachea, curved convex laterally. Typical appearance of achalasia of the cardia; the thickened oesophageal walls can be seen in the root of the neck and the speckled appearance is due to food residues. The diagnosis is easily proven by barium meal (see Plate 2.30). Vertical streaks over the heart shadow are artefacts.

Plate 2.29   Calcification within the heart shadow along its left border and apex; the heart shape itself is unusually triangular. Lateral view (see Plate 2.32) shows that the calcification extends all round the heart − typical appearances of calcified pericardium of constrictive pericarditis. (The heart shape may be much more bizarre than this in some cases.)

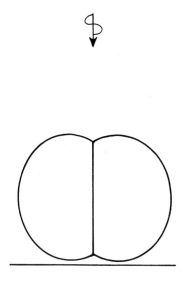

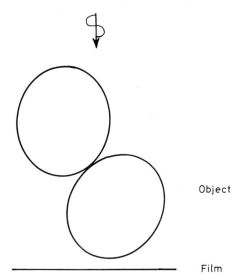

Object

Film

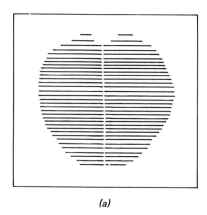

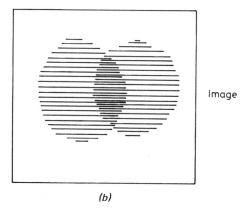

Image

(a)   (b)

The heart borders

It should be noted whether or not the heart borders are sharp or blurred, for a number of deductions may be made from this observation.

It is convenient at this point to describe the theory underlying the 'outline signs'* by which the broncho-pulmonary segments may be identified in PA films of the chest, for the principles involved are of wide general application in diagnostic radiology.

If, as in *Figure 2.3,* two objects or masses of similar radiographic density (for example, of water density) are radiographed side by side, close together, no boundary or border will be seen

* Sometimes called 'silhouette signs'.

Figure 2.3   Diagram showing the images produced (a) when two objects of similar radiographic density are radiographed side in contact, no line of demarcation being seen on the image, and (b) when two objects overlap, one behind the other, when their outlines are visible on the resulting radiograph.

between them. The simplest example of this is the lack of border between the shadows of the liver and the heart on the normal chest film. If, on the other hand, one of the objects or masses lies behind the other then a border will be visible on the image where one overlaps the other, since there are two thicknesses in the region of overlap and only one beyond it. If this principle is applied

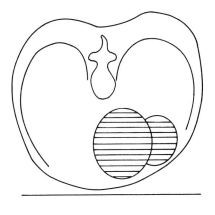
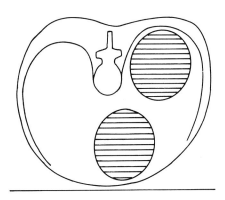

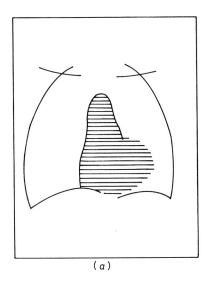
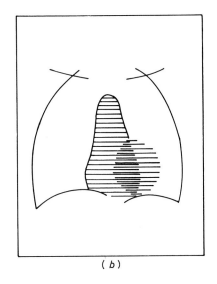

(a)   (b)

Figure 2.4   Diagram showing that a patch of consolidation or other lesion of water density, lying (a) against the heart shadow produces an image in which the heart border is lost, and (b) behind the heart shadow when it produces an image in which the heart border is preserved (compare with Figure 2.3).

to the chest, as seen diagrammatically in transverse section in *Figure 2.4*, it is clear that the shadow of a mass of water density lying alongside the heart will not be separable from the heart shadow, the border of which will vanish; whereas if it lies behind the heart the border of the heart shadow will be visible, superimposed on the shadow of the mass. Similar reasoning may also be applied to

masses lying against the diaphragm and, of course, to fluid in the pleural cavity, when the diaphragmatic outline disappears. This principle of the 'outline sign' can be applied in the chest to the localization in the PA view of pneumonic consolidations in the broncho-pulmonary segments.

The anatomy is important. The lungs are divided into upper and lower lobes by the oblique fissure on both sides which run downwards and forwards from the region of the 4th rib posteriorly to the diaphragm, and twist inwards as they do so like an aeroplane propeller so that they are parallel to the coronal plane above and lie obliquely, somewhere between the coronal and sagittal planes, on reaching the diaphragm. The actual point of contact with the diaphragm on either

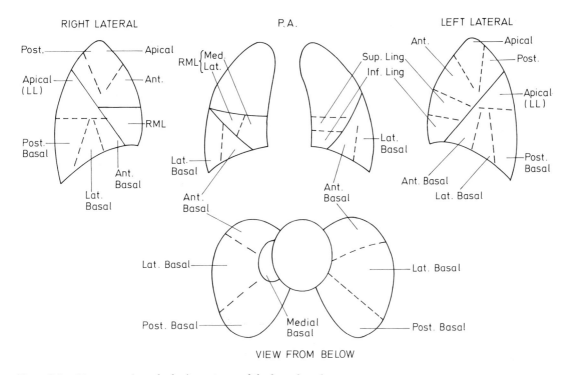

Figure 2.5 Diagram to show the basic anatomy of the bronchopulmonary segments.
Upper lobes: Apical–apical segment; Post.–posterior segment; Ant.–anterior segment.
Lower lobes: Apical (LL)–apical segment, lower lobe; Post. basal–posterior basal segment; Lat. basal–lateral basal
segment; Ant. basal–anterior basal segment.
Right middle lobe: Med. (RML)–medial segment, right middle lobe; Lat. (RML)–lateral segment, right middle lobe.
Left upper lobe: Sup. ling–superior lingular segment; Inf. ling–inferior lingular segment.
Right lower lobe: Med. basal–medial basal segment, right lower lobe.

side is rather variable – almost anywhere from the heart border to the costo-phrenic angle – but usually, in PA view, in the medial third of the diaphragmatic outline and in lateral view the cardiophrenic angle.

The right middle lobe is bounded above by the right horizontal fissure which runs from the heart border at the level of the anterior end of the right 4th rib to meet the right 6th rib (usually) in the mid-axillary line, and below and behind by the oblique fissure; on the left the corresponding part of the lung is the lingula of the upper lobe.

The lobes are further divided into segments: anterior, apical and posterior in the right upper lobe, lateral and medial in the right middle lobe, and apical, anterior basal, lateral basal and posterior basal in the right lower lobe plus a small medial basal or paracardiac segment. In the left upper lobe, there are similarly anterior, apical and posterior segments plus the two segments of the

lingula, superior and inferior lingular segments. (Strictly speaking, the apical and posterior segments are parts of one apico-posterior segment.) The left lower lobe has apical, anterior basal, lateral basal and posterior basal segments only. These are shown diagrammatically in *Figure 2.5.*

Bearing in mind this anatomy, it has proved possible to construct a logical scheme making use of the 'outline signs' to locate consolidations in the various segments on a PA view and this scheme is shown diagrammatically in *Figure 2.6.* The lateral views are also shown and are, of course, valuable in confirmation of the location but it is possible to locate the segments without their aid in most cases. Some additional comment is necessary. Upper lobe apical shadowing is never visible in lateral view because the shoulders get in the way, and for this reason no lateral view has been shown in the diagram of these segments. It will be noted that posterior segmental consolidation in

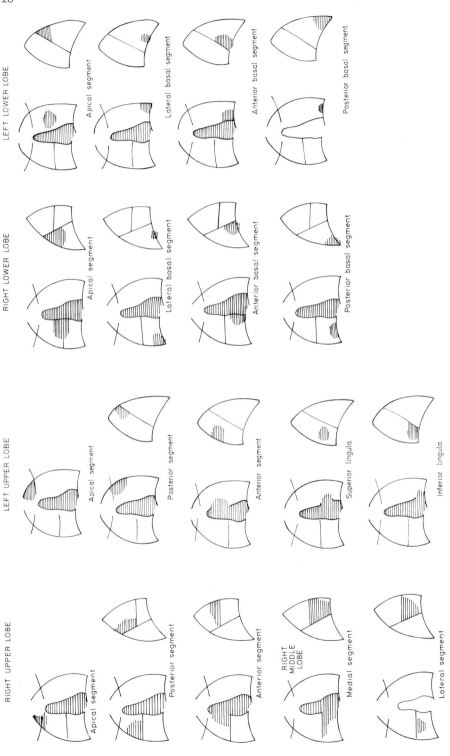

Figure 2.6   Diagram of a scheme by which segmental consolidation in the lung may be located in a plain PA film, making use of the 'outline' signs. Note loss of outline of the right heart border from consolidations of anterior segment, right upper lobe and medial segment, right middle lobe, of the left heart border from anterior segments, and superior and inferior lingular segments of the left upper lobe and of the diaphragm from lateral anterior basal segments of both lower lobes. Note that the heart border is clear in a consolidation of apical segment of either lower lobe and posterior segment of either upper lobe, and the diaphragmatic border clear in an isolated consolidation of the posterior basal segment of either lower lobe.

the right upper lobe tends to lie slightly more laterally, with a clear zone separating it from the heart, whereas anterior segmental consolidation is slightly more medial and always blurs the heart border. Both are limited below by the horizontal fissure, but because the fissure may not be plane but curved, some part of the consolidation in an anterior segment may appear below the line taken to represent the fissure.

Infection in the right middle lobe blurs the lower part of the right heart border unless the lateral segment only is involved. Right middle lobe consolidation is always limited above by the horizontal fissure. On the left, blurring of the heart border may be due to consolidation of, from above downwards, the anterior segment of the upper lobe, superior lingula and inferior lingula.

On the other hand, segmental consolidations in the lower lobe, being posterior, leave the heart borders clear and this in particular serves to distinguish the apical segment of the lower lobe from both the anterior segment of the upper lobe and from the right middle lobe and lingula, all of which blur the heart border. The basal segments, however, blur the diaphragm when consolidated — the anterior basal segment in its medial two-thirds, and the lateral basal segment in its lateral third. The posterior basal segment of the lower lobe blurs the posterior third of the diaphragm in lateral view but this is not visible in the PA view and such a consolidation alone is merely seen as a shadow in the lung base with the diaphragm dome superimposed upon it.

Segments may consolidate singly or in combination, usually consistent with accumulation of secretions in dependent bronchial branches. All the basal segments of a lower lobe, sparing the apical segment, may be consolidated at once, or the posterior basal and apical segments, or lingular and left posterior basal segments, for example.

It should be added that there is usually some element of collapse in most consolidations, and an element of consolidation is present in most cases of collapse of lung, so that collapse of a lobe or a segment presents exactly the same sort of outline signs although the extent of the dense shadow is obviously less in a pure collapse.

The importance of identifying the location of a consolidation lies in the manner in which postural drainage can be performed, ensuring that a position can be adopted during the various manoeuvres undertaken by the physiotherapist so that the sputum can drain vertically out of the relevant bronchial branch. If, in fact, the lesion proves to be more sinister than a simple infective lesion (for example, underlying carcinoma or, more fortunately, a bronchial adenoma or foreign body) and surgery is contemplated, its location is clearly of paramount importance. On the other hand, if a lung lesion does not show the expected anatomical pattern of segmental or lobar consolidation, then it must be something else.

Now, having in mind the diagrams in *Figure 2.6*, look at the PA x-ray films reproduced in *Plates 2.33–2.40* and try to identify the segments involved. Then turn to the lateral views (*Plates 2.41–2.48*), and see if they confirm your predictions.

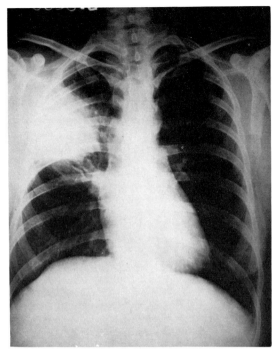

Plate 2.33

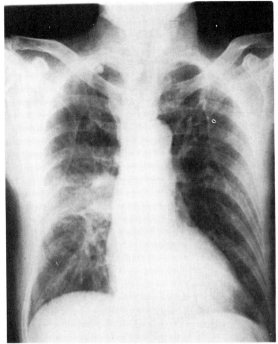

Plate 2.34

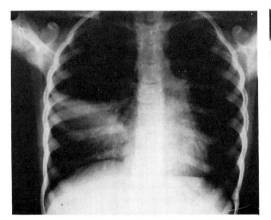

Plate 2.35

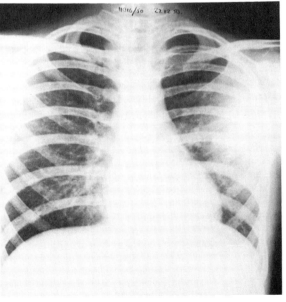

Plate 2.36

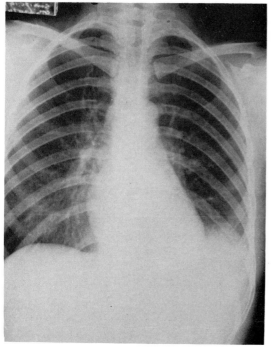

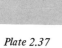

Plate 2.37

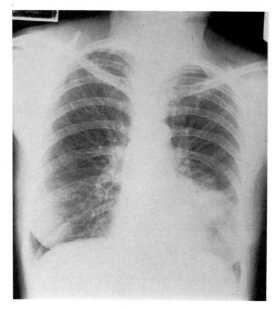

Plate 2.38

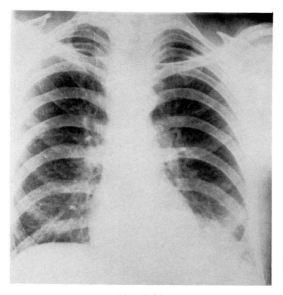

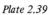

Plate 2.39

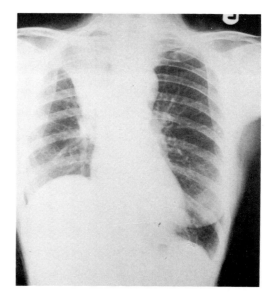

Plate 2.40

SOLUTIONS

Plate 2.33   Patch of consolidation on the right, bounded below by the horizontal fissure medially by the rib cage and clear of the right heart border which is clearly defined. The apex of the lung is normal. This is therefore in the posterior segment of the upper lobe. The lateral view (Plate 2.41) confirms this; note that there is some extension forwards on to the horizontal fissure.

Plate 2.34   Patch of consolidation in the right mid-zone, with poorly defined upper and lower borders but associated with a clear right heart border; this must be posterior and in the apical segment of the right lower lobe. This is confirmed in lateral view (Plate 2.42).

Plate 2.35   Patch of consolidation in the right mid-zone with a sharp upper border, presumably the horizontal fissure, indistinguishable medially from the heart shadow, the right heart border being lost, and having a poorly defined lower border which rises as it passes laterally; the diaphragmatic outline is clear. This is the typical appearance of consolidation of the right middle lobe, which is confirmed in the lateral view (Plate 2.43). Note also that there is some blurring of the left heart border, suggesting that there is some involvement of the lingula also.

Plate 2.36   Patch of consolidation in the left mid-zone, lying against the rib cage with poorly defined upper and lower borders and clear of the left heart border which is well defined. This must be in the posterior segment of the left upper lobe, differing only from the right in lacking a horizontal fissure to give a straight lower border (compare with Plate 2.33). Lateral view confirms (Plate 2.44).

Plate 2.37   Dense consolidation at the left base with loss of the diaphragmatic outline but preservation of the left heart border. Typical appearances of consolidation of the left lower lobe, sparing the apical segment; lateral view (Plate 2.45) confirms and also shows loss of the diaphragmatic outline.

Plate 2.38   Patch of consolidation blurring the middle part of the left heart border though the lowest part is clear; this must be in the superior lingular segment, evident in lateral view (Plate 2.46).

Plate 2.39   Patch of consolidation at the left base through which the diaphragmatic outline can be seen and also the heart border except at its extreme lower part. This should suggest consolidation of the inferior lingula plus the posterior basal segment, as confirmed in lateral view (Plate 2.47).

Plate 2.40   Dense shadow to the right of the superior mediastinum, obscuring its right border. The horizontal fissure is not visible in its normal position but the right infero-lateral border of the shadow is sharp and concave downwards and represents the raised fissure. The right hilum looks enlarged; this is the classical appearance of collapse of the right upper lobe due to an obstructing neoplasm in the hilum. It is just possible to make out a transradiancy representing the trachea displaced to the right below the clavicle. Lateral view (Plate 2.48) confirms the enlarged hilum and the wedge-shaped collapsed upper lobe, the oblique fissure having moved upwards and forwards in addition.

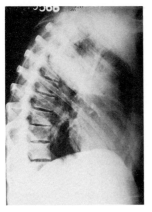

Plate 2.41

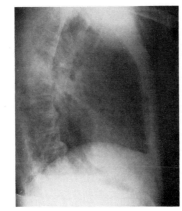

Plate 2.42

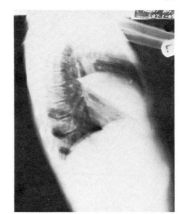

Plate 2.43

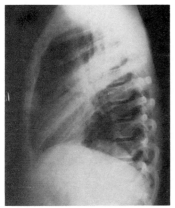

Plate 2.44

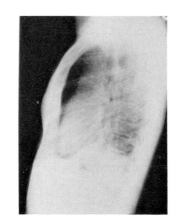

Plate 2.45

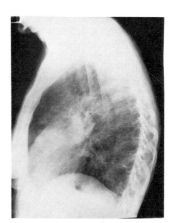

Plate 2.46

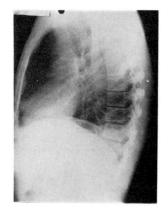

Plate 2.47

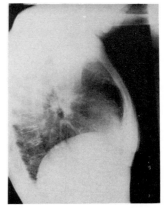

Plate 2.48

THE HILA

The hila of the lungs consist normally of main bronchi and their upper and lower lobe branches, pulmonary arteries and veins and lymphatic vessels and glands. Most of the shadow appears to be made up of the pulmonary arteries with the upper pulmonary veins superimposed, their tributaries accompanying the arterial branches. The lower lobe veins tend to be more horizontal and in the lower part of the hilum. The differences in distribution of the arteries and veins are shown in *Figures 2.7* and *2.8*. The pulmonary arteries sweep backwards up and over the main bronchi, giving off upper lobe branches before turning downwards. It should be noted that normally the lateral margins are *concave*, between the upward and the downward sweep of the upper and lower lobe vessels; although a middle vessel can usually be seen as well, this does not alter the general

Shape

If the normal concavity is absent then the hilum is abnormal. Usually a convexity indicates either an enlarged gland or an enlarged pulmonary artery.

Size

An attempt should be made to consider whether the hila are larger than normal.

ENLARGED GLANDS

Enlarged glands may be due to inflammatory disease — simple infections in children, tuberculosis at any age, or sarcoid are the commonest. Hilar glands in sarcoidosis are usually (though not

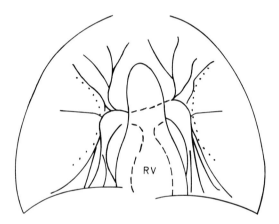

Figure 2.7 Diagram to show the general layout of the pulmonary arteries and their main branches. The interrupted line lateral to each hilum illustrates the concave shape to be noted in the normal.

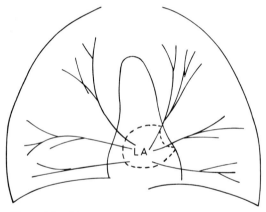

Figure 2.8 Diagram to show the general layout of the pulmonary veins. This should be compared with Figure 2.7. Note that the upper lobe veins parallel the course of the upper lobe arteries closely but the lower lobe veins are nearly horizontal and thus cross the arteries almost at right angles.

shape. This normal appearance and that of the branching vessels leading out into the lung fields should always be specifically looked for, remember that altogether they carry as much blood as the aorta — 5 litres a minute in the adult — so they have normally an appreciable volume and it is worth turning back to the normal chest shown in *Figure 1.2a* to notice this. The points to be looked for in the systematic scrutiny are the shape, height and size of the hila and the size and distribution of the vessels.

always) lobulated and symmetrical and often accompanied by nodular shadowing in the lung fields. Enlarged hilar glands may also be due to neoplasm, either secondary to lung or other neoplasm or primary as in a reticulosis (for example, a lymphoma such as Hodgkin's disease, lymphosarcoma, lymphatic leukemia or the like). An asymmetry is much more likely here. Whatever the cause, enlarged glands in the hilum frequently show a lobulated outline, and this is very useful in distinguishing them from enlarged vessels. The appearance may be complicated by a medially placed mass in the lung which partly overlies the hilum, and a lateral view is most useful in identifying this situation. It also helps in distinguishing glands from pulmonary artery since the glands often lie below the level of the carina, whereas the main mass of the pulmonary artery normally lies above it.

Calcified hilar glands are usually due to healed tuberculosis but are sometimes seen in occupational disease.

ENLARGED PULMONARY ARTERIES

Enlarged pulmonary arteries occur mainly in two groups of conditions: in congenital heart disease with left to right shunt (increased flow) or post-stenotic dilatation, and in peripheral lung disease

The commoner causes of hilar enlargement are summarized in *Figure 2.9*.

Height
Any variation in the normal heights of the hila and their relationships to each other should be noted. Collapse or fibrosis of all or part of the upper lobe will elevate the hilum on that side, and of the lower lobe will lower it; partial or complete lobectomy has a similar effect. It should be recalled that the left hilum normally lies higher than the right by a distance which is somewhere between the width of a rib and a rib space, and any alteration in this relationship must be regarded as abnormal.

Size of vessels
The appearance of the branches of the pulmonary arteries is frequently most valuable. In a left to

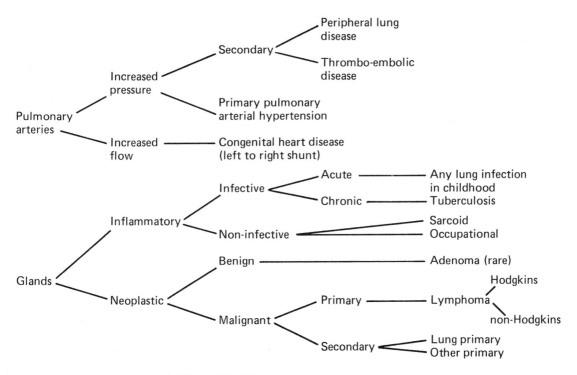

Figure 2.9   Common causes of hilar enlargement.

and other causes of pulmonary arterial hypertension. In both cases there is usually some alteration of heart shape with right ventricular enlargement and prominence of the pulmonary conus.

right shunt they are all enlarged, whereas in pulmonary arterial hypertension and long-standing peripheral lung disease the peripheral branches are much smaller, both absolutely and in comparison, although the main pulmonary arteries are large. When hilar enlargement is due to glands, the vessels are of course normal. If the upper lobe vessels alone are enlarged (they are said to resemble an upturned moustache) the likelihood is that these are engorged veins; this is seen in the pulmonary venous hypertension of mitral stenosis and in various forms of acute left heart failure, including cardiac infarction, usually associated with horizontal septal lines near the costophrenic angles (*see* under 'Linear shadows'). Sometimes the horizontal lower lobe pulmonary veins are visible when engorged.

The azygos vein, usually indistinguishable, is occasionally seen end-on in the angle between the trachea and the right main bronchus; if it has failed to pass medial to the lung during development but 'scythes' down through the apex, as it were, an azygos fissure may be seen.

Distribution of vessels

Alteration in the customary distribution of the lung vessels may be produced by the same factors which displace hila — fibrosis and shrinkage, collapse or lobectomy — and also by emphysematous bullae and space-occupying masses. In the absence of any of these, disappearance of a particular vessel, either by comparison with the opposite side or with a previous normal film, is sometimes the only visible intimation of a pulmonary embolus.

Bearing the foregoing in mind, the hilar shadows and pulmonary vessels of the x-ray films shown in *Plates 2.49–2.57* should be inspected, after a look at the soft tissues, the bony cage and the central shadow. On some of the films there is more than one abnormality which, taken together, suggest a definite diagnosis.

38

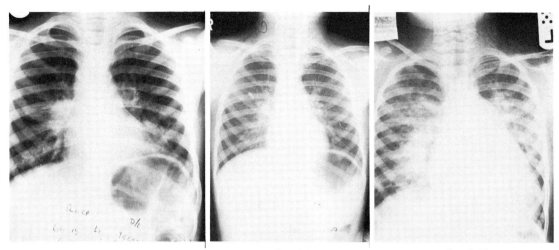

Plate 2.49   *Plate 2.50*   *Plate 2.51*

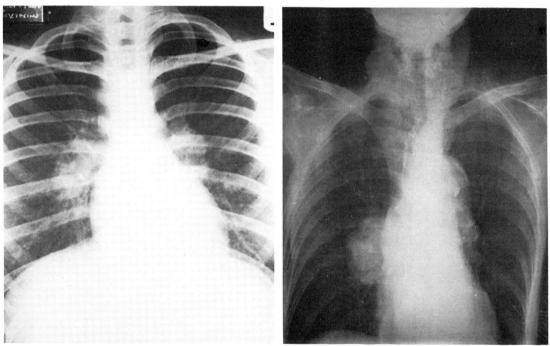

Plate 2.52   *Plate 2.53*

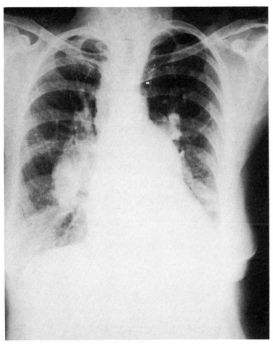

Plate 2.54

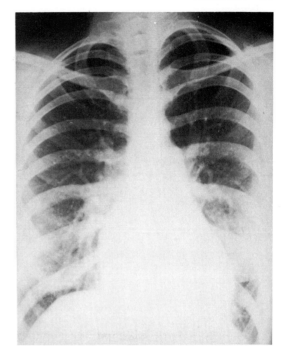

Plate 2.55

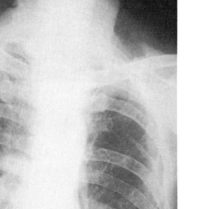

Plate 2.56

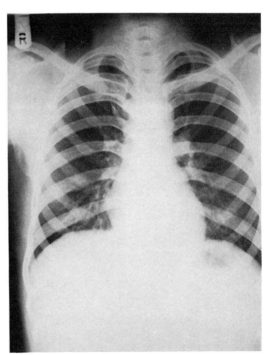

Plate 2.57

SOLUTIONS

Plate 2.49   Both hila are enlarged, with an irregular outline, and there is some patchy consolidation in the inferior lingula. Typical appearances of primary tuberculosis in a child, primary focus in the lingula and the hilar glands enlarging secondarily.

Plate 2.50   Healed calcified tuberculous primary complex in a well-nourished child aged 4 years.

Plate 2.51   Child's heart is enlarged due to RV+ with prominent pulmonary conus, enlarged pulmonary arteries and a well-marked pulmonary plethora. Ventricular septal defect with left to right shunt.

Plate 2.52   Bilateral, symmetrical, lobulated hilar enlargement, typical of enlarged glands. Even in the absence of abnormalities in the lung pattern, this is most likely to be sarcoid.

Plate 2.53   Lobulated enlargement of the right hilum, the left being normal. This is most likely to be neoplastic, probably a central lung carcinoma with hilar glands.

Plate 2.54   Massively enlarged hilar shadows on both sides. On the right an upper lobe vessel is continuous with the shadow and on the left large vessels can be seen end-on as part of it, but the remainder of the hilum is concealed by a greatly enlarged pulmonary conus, and the whole heart is enlarged. Peripheral vessels are relatively poorly shown. This is typical of a long-standing left to right shunt with right ventricular enlargement and some degree of pulmonary hypertension. (Atrial septal defect at the age of 77 years.)

Plate 2.55   Prominent pulmonary arteries on both sides with a prominent pulmonary conus and enlarged right ventricle; atrial septal defect in a young woman.

Plate 2.56   Normal right hilum, but on the left there is only a single stretched vessel. The left 5th rib shows the typical appearance of regeneration after subperiosteal resection for thoracotomy, so there has presumably been a lobectomy. A small round opacity in the right upper zone may well be a secondary deposit, suggesting neoplasm as the original aetiology.

Plate 2.57   Normal hilar shadows, but there is an azygos fissure and the azygos vein can be seen above and lateral to the right hilum.

THE LUNG FIELDS

The lung fields are the part of the chest film considered by many to be all that matters; all too frequently, it is all that is looked at, with perhaps a glance at the heart shadow. Initial scrutiny of other areas of the chest — soft tissues, bones, central shadow and hila and lung vessels — may well prove rewarding in that the mind will be primed for possibilities in the lung fields. If all other appearances are normal, at least they can be removed from the scene, as it were, and the ribs should not confuse the lung pattern nor the costal cartilages the hila. One's eye should not immediately fix on what appears to be an abnormal shadow and imagine that it must, if correctly interpreted, give the complete answer; it may well only serve to distract the attention from a feature which is, in fact, much more significant. It is necessary to look systematically at the lung fields and the following routine is suggested: (1) pleura; (2) horizontal and other fissures; (3) compare rib spaces; (4) peripheral lung pattern; and (5) abnormal shadows.

Pleura

Look all round the edges of both lung fields, starting at the apex, down the lateral chest walls to the costophrenic angles, along the diaphragms and up the borders of the central shadow to the apices (central shadow and diaphragms should already have been noted). There is normally a thin linear shadow just beneath the first rib (rarely the second also) and occasionally just medial to the lower thoracic wall laterally. These are known as 'companion shadows' and are of no significance. Rather thicker shadows over the tops of the apices usually represent old pleural thickening due to healed subclinical tuberculosis. Thickening of this sort, however, on the lower lateral thoracic wall, particularly if uneven and in plaques, is seen in asbestosis; and an oval or rounded prominence may be due to an associated mesothelioma. If the diaphragm looks straight and is elevated laterally this is probably due to an old adhesion from previous effusion or empyema; the lesser degrees of this may produce only a 'rounding off' of the costophrenic angle. This has to be distinguished from the normal step-like appearance of the slips of origin of the diaphragm seen on a very deep inspiration and sometimes in emphysema.

Sometimes pleural thickening is extensive but it is usually in one or more plaques with a clearly defined border (it is often the result of an encysted effusion); these do not correspond to any unexpected distribution in the lung. They are sometimes calcified, producing bizarre appearances which are usually easily recognizable.

AIR IN THE PLEURA

If there is air in the pleura (pneumothorax) scrutiny of the region just inside the thoracic wall shows an absence of vascular markings which, if followed inwards, leads to the fine linear shadow of the lung edge — easily confused with or masked by the cortex of a rib towards the apex or in the upper zone, although it is easier to identify as it runs across the rib shadows down the lateral border of the lung. The lung edge can also be seen sometimes above the diaphragm, and in the later phase of recovery (say, 8th to 16th day) medial to the lung, slightly separated from the mediastinum (paracardiac line). The latter may, occasionally, be the only clue to the diagnosis. If the pneumothorax is extensive and there is appreciable collapse of the lung, a large transradiant area will be seen and the lung may occupy only a small area of the hemithorax; in such cases part or all of a lobe is sometimes opaque. It is important to note that in most cases the lung remains transradiant. Rarely, part of the lung is held out and fails to collapse because it is stuck to the chest wall by a pleural adhesion.

FLUID IN THE PLEURA

Fluid in the pleura (pleural effusion), being of water density, produces a dense white shadow; if the effusion is extensive, the hemithorax undergoes a virtual 'white-out'*. Having the same radiographic density as solid organs, it abolishes the diaphragmatic outline, including the costophrenic angle. Indeed, in a very small effusion, all that may be seen is an apparent rounding off or loss of the costophrenic angle. As the effusion gets larger, it appears to rise up the lateral wall of the hemithorax, but this is largely a false appearance. The effect is best explained by considering the type of glass tumbler shown in *Figure 2.10a*. It is obvious that the glass is the same thickness all round at any given level but the thickness is only perceptible at the sides where it is seen end-on. Similarly, if a rubber ball is pushed

*The appearances are the same whether the fluid is a simple effusion, blood or pus as in an empyema.

down into a container of water, the water will rise at the sides as it is displaced from the centre, and a radiograph of this would show a similar appearance (*Figure 2.10b*). In the same way the lung, floating in the fluid of a pleural effusion, is surrounded by the same thickness of fluid all round but it is only obvious at the sides. It appears to be higher laterally in a moderately sized effusion, but this is because the heart, lying anteriorly, conceals the fluid lying against the spine, and the heart border is preserved because only a small thickness of fluid lies alongside it; also, the presence of the hilum prevents displacement of the medial part of the lung by the fluid. In a large effusion, the heart

occur, or a broncho-pleural fistula, there will be a gas-fluid level — a clearly defined upper limit to the fluid. This is mobile, as can be shown by taking a film with the patient lying on his side.

Horizontal and other fissures

The oblique fissure on either side is not usually seen in a PA view but an effusion in it, encysted or otherwise, may produce an ill-defined shadow in the lung field; sometimes confusing in heart failure. It is often lozenge-shaped in a lateral view. Pleural thickening in the lower end of the oblique fissure is common and produces the

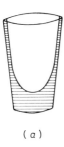 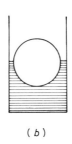 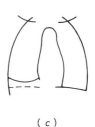 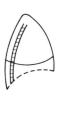

(*a*)   (*b*)   (*c*)   (*d*)

Figure 2.10   Diagrams to illustrate by analogies the radiological appearance of a pleural effusion. In (a) is represented a common type of glass tumbler with a relatively thick bottom; by transmitted light the sides of the glass are only seen 'end-on' at the sides but are clearly the same thickness all round. In (b) a ball is pushed downwards into a cylinder containing water which rises up all round the ball at the sides, but would produce the appearance shown if radiographed. (c) and (d) Illustrating the appearances in PA and lateral views of the chest; note that the medial part of the effusion is partly concealed behind the heart border, giving rise to the impression that the effusion only rises on the lateral aspect.

border disappears and fluid may sometimes even be seen over the lung apex. When the patient is horizontal (for example, in a supine chest film) the effusion, being fluid and therefore moving about with gravity, is posterior and is only represented by a narrow shadow all round the lung edges, but there is a general loss of transradiancy and the lung looks generally more dense — a confusing picture until the mechanism is appreciated.

If both air and fluid are present (hydropneumothorax), for example, after tapping a pleural effusion when some air may accidentally have entered, in penetrating injuries of the chest, sometimes in the course of a simple pneumothorax when a small amount of bleeding may

appearance which has been incorrectly termed 'tenting of the diaphragm' though it is a good visual description.

The horizontal fissure on the right normally reaches the 6th rib in the mid-axillary line, crossing the anterior end of the right 4th rib. If it is markedly raised and bowed upwards, loss of volume in the right upper lobe is suggested (fibrosis or collapse). If lowered, it is not usually visible since right middle lobe collapse is commonly the cause and the associated opacity usually conceals and includes the fissure. Elevation of the right diaphragm usually raises the fissure but not when it is due to a basal lung infarct (because of the loss of volume) — a useful differential point.

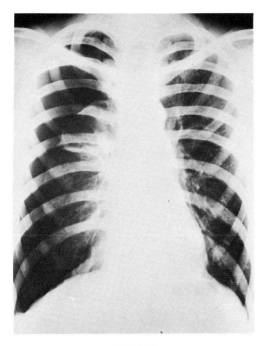
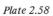

Plate 2.58

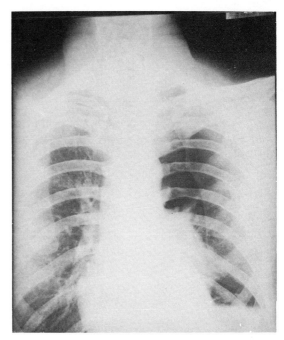

Plate 2.59

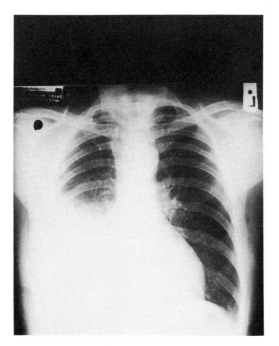

Plate 2.60

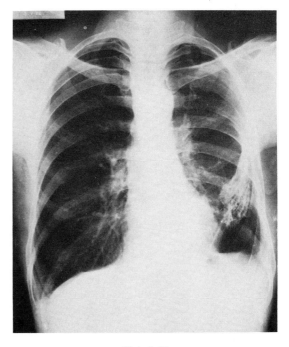

Plate 2.61

SOLUTIONS

Plate 2.58   Right pneumothorax. There are no lung markings in the periphery of the right hemithorax; the lung edge is visible, and there is some collapse of the medial part of the lung.

Plate 2.60   The lower part of the right hemithorax is opaque, the diaphragm and the right heart border are not visible, and the upper margin of the opacity is concave and ill-defined — typical appearances of a pleural effusion (compare with Plate 2.37). Less easy to see is the right breast shadow, the left being absent; old left mastectomy, with metastases involving the right pleura.

Plate 2.59   Left hydropneumothorax. In addition to the signs of pneumothorax, there is also an air−fluid level in the left lower zone.

Plate 2.61   Bizarre and irregular partly calcified shadow in the right middle and lower zones — typical appearance of a calcified pleural plaque. Below it there is a transradiant region with no lung markings and a flattened diaphragm with adhesions; this is probably an encysted pneumothorax.

Rib spaces

It is now time to inspect the lung fields in detail. The first step is to scan from side to side, from above downwards, comparing the appearances of the lung fields as seen between the anterior rib spaces. Above the anterior part of the 1st rib is usually called the apex of the lung. Between the 1st and 3rd ribs is the upper zone, 3rd and 5th ribs the mid-zone, and from the 5th ribs downwards the lower zone. If the soft tissues and rib cage have already been considered there should not be too much to do at this stage other than to assess whether or not there are variations between the two sides, and between the different parts of the lung fields, whether they are uniformly normal or uniformly abnormal. The distribution of any lesions noted should be observed. A pneumothorax, if missed at the first inspection of the pleura, may be spotted now as may also a soft-tissue defect.

Peripheral lung pattern

Normal peripheral lung contains only alveoli and bronchioles containing air, fine blood vessels and relatively little stroma. Consequently, the branching and progressively narrowing vascular pattern is all that should be seen in the normal chest film. This lung pattern may become abnormal in two principal ways. The blood vessels may be increased in size and number, or decreased, as already described; and the lung tissue itself may become radio-opaque and thus visible on the film, or may appear more transradiant than usual.

INCREASED TRANSRADIANCY

Increased transradiancy, if associated with either a distorted vascular pattern due to localized bullae, or a generalized or localized loss of peripheral pulmonary arterial pattern, may be due to emphysema, but it is important not to make such a diagnosis without good evidence of lung destruction. It may be mimicked by chronic obstructive bronchitis. The secondary signs commonly ascribed to emphysema, that is, low flat diaphragms exposing the anterior ends of the 7th ribs and an expanded upper rib cage, also occur in severe asthma and occasionally in normal people. Localized loss of lung vascular pattern is sometimes seen in pulmonary embolism but with slight increase in transradiancy. Obstructive or 'ball-valve' emphysema due to foreign body, tuberculous glands in children, or neoplasm in a main bronchial branch may be confusing; the expanded and relatively transradiant lung produces a mediastinal displacement away from the affected side, which may be mistaken for a displacement towards the relatively more radio-opaque normal side, thought to be collapsed. The differentiation may be made by taking an expiratory film. In obstructive emphysema the mediastinum moves towards the normal side in expiration as that lung empties; in a collapse there is slight movement in the reverse direction or no movement at all. Unilateral hypertransradiancy of one lung (McCleod's syndrome) without mediastinal shift to the opposite side is usually due to obliterative bronchiolitis but the rare pulmonary artery hypoplasia can produce a similar appearance.

INCREASED OPACITY

Increased opacity of the lung tissue may take the form of one or more discrete shadows, or the appearance of a background pattern in addition to the vascular pattern.

Background patterns

The interpretation of background patterns is one of the most difficult tasks in chest radiology and is fraught with misconceptions, hazards and traps for the unwary. Some can be recognized but others are completely non-specific and occur in a variety of conditions. A classification of the appearances, however, will at least assist in narrowing the search for a solution into groups of possibilities. If an abnormal lung pattern is present, the following questions should be posed.

(1) What is the distribution of the abnormality? Is it unilateral, bilateral, widespread, apical, basal, segmental or confined to the mid-zones?

(2) Is it composed of:

  (a) Nodules (nodular shadowing)?

  (b) Lines (linear shadows, or a network, that is, reticulation)?

  (c) Ring shadows?

  (d) Mixtures of the above?

(3) If nodular, are the nodules:

  (a) Under or over 2 mm in diameter?

  (b) Dense ('hard') or less dense ('soft')?

  (c) Well-defined with sharp edges or ill-defined with blurred edges, even coalescent?

(4) If linear, are the lines:

  (a) Anatomical (for example, fissures, vessels)?

  (b) Radial?

  (c) Horizontal?

  (d) Reticular?

(5) If ring shadows, are they:

(*a*) Small (under 2 mm diameter), medium or large (over 1 cm in diameter)?

(*b*) If small, are they to true circular structures or lesions or to airspaces amongst a network of pathological tissue?

(*c*) Medium or large, thin-walled or thick-walled?

(*d*) Smooth and well-defined, irregular or ill-defined, in their interior and exterior walls?

(6) Is there any other evidence on the film which would assist in making the diagnosis, for example, change in heart size or shape, enlarged lymph glands?

This classification of pathological lung patterns is diagrammatically illustrated in *Figure 2.11*.

DISTRIBUTION

An abnormal pattern largely confined to the lower zones is common in congestive cardiac failure (usually bilateral), bronchopneumonia (one or both sides), in idiopathic pulmonary fibrosis, bronchiectasis and asbestosis. Mid-zone involvement is seen in those types of pulmonary oedema associated with acute left ventricular failure ('batswing shadows') and mid-zone and upper-zone distribution is usual in silicosis and coal pneumoconiosis. Apical and upper-zone predominance is usual in localized tuberculous and fungous infections. In the absence of a characteristic distribution, other evidence will be required.

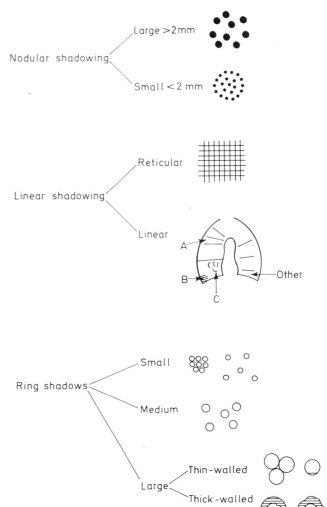

Figure 2.11   Diagram to illustrate the different types of lung background pattern to be looked for in the lung fields.

NODULAR SHADOWING

Soft, often coalescent, ill-defined nodular shadow-ing of varying sizes up to 4 mm, most marked at the bases, is seen in congestive cardiac failure, due to alveolar oedema. This is often associated with pleural effusions of varying sizes (often quite small) or with short, fine, horizontal, septal lines in the costophrenic angles (lines 'B' of Kerley, of which more anon), enlarged upper-lobe pul-monary veins and an enlarged heart. If extensive pulmonary oedema is present there may be rather larger patches of fluffy appearance, seen also in

or of certain fumes and gases and falls into one of three groups.

(1) Non-fibrogenic, due to inert dusts which produce negligible pathological reaction in the lungs. The particles themselves are radio-opaque and produce widespread, dense, well-defined nodular shadows, 0.5–3 mm in size, associated with similarly dense hilar glands. Examples are iron oxide in arc welders and iron foundry workers (siderosis), and tin ore dust and oxide fumes in tin refiners (stannosis).

(2) Granulomatous, due to beryllium and its compounds, some fungal spores (for example,

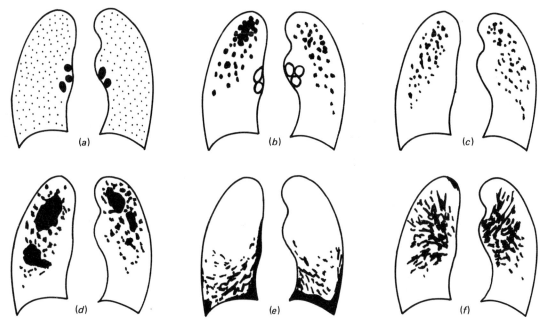

Figure 2.12 Occupational lung disease. (a) Siderosis, stannosis, etc.; dense hilar nodes. (b) Nodular silicosis with mass in right upper zone and peripherally calcified hilar nodes. (c) Coal pneumoconiosis – early stage. (d) Coal pneumo-coniosis – PMF. (e) Asbestosis. (f) Chronic extrinsic allergic alveolitis.

acute heart failure, drowning and other aspiration effects, including acute heroin, barbiturate and similar poisoning.

Generalized nodular shadowing, soft but reasonably well defined and up to 2 mm in size, is commonly due to one of four main groups of conditions,. namely, occupational disease, sar-coidosis, miliary tuberculosis and miliary carcino-matosis. There are numerous other causes, but they can nearly all be associated with one of these four.

Occupational lung disease is due to inhalation of mineral or organic dusts (the pneumoconioses)

M.faeni in farmers' lung) and the proteins in certain bird droppings (bird fancier's lung). Here, local reaction in the lung produces widespread, less dense, poorly defined nodules, 1–5 mm in size. Disease due to such organic dusts is known as extrinsic allergic alveolitis, and is usually in the upper halves of the lung fields.

(3) Fibrogenic, in which the particles excite a collagenous fibrosis. In silicosis and coal miners' pneumoconiosis they appear as discrete nodular shadows of moderate density, from less than 1 mm up to 5 mm, mostly in the upper and mid-zones. Linear shadows (*vide infra*) are often present.

Hilar glands with calcified edges may be seen. Later, the disease progresses and the large, bilateral, roughly rounded opacities of 'progressive massive fibrosis' may appear in coal pneumoconiosis. In asbestosis the opacities are finely or coarsely irregular and predominant in the lower zones, often associated with pleural thickening.

In *Figure 2.12* the typical pattern and distribution of different types of pneumoconiosis are illustrated.

In sarcoidosis the nodular appearance is due to widespread, small, granulomatous lesions. It may show as an almost reticular appearance or range up to larger blotches. Bilateral, symmetrical, hilar, glandular enlargement is common though not always present at the same time. If the disease does not resolve spontaneously or in response to treatment it may progress to severe fibrosis. Included here should be other conditions of poorly understood aetiology or pathogenesis producing similar fine nodular shadows such as cryptogenic fibrosing alveolitis, rheumatoid and liver disease and scleroderma.

Miliary tuberculosis in children or adults produces a widespread 'snowstorm' appearance throughout the lungs. There may be large mediastinal or hilar glands or evidence of active tuberculosis, but often these are absent. Somewhat similar appearances may be produced by other infections such as miliary bronchopneumonia and miliary fungous infections, including acute histoplasmosis.

Miliary carcinomatosis may be indistinguishable from any of the moderately dense patterns, but there are commonly repeated blood-borne showers of small metastases so that the distinguishing feature is nodules of differing sizes.

Well-defined, basal, nodular shadows, which may be calcified and even ossified, are a feature of long-standing mitral stenosis but they are sometimes more widely distributed; here the heart shape and size and distribution of lung vessels may help in the differential diagnosis.

Calcified nodular shadows scattered through the lung, if relatively evenly spaced, are likely to be due to a previous attack of chickenpox in adult life or to old histoplasmosis; if in one or two irregular clusters, more in the upper zones, they are likely to be due to old tuberculosis, healed miliary tuberculosis calcifies.

Widespread nodular shadows of different sizes are almost always due to repeated blood-borne showers of secondary carcinoma or sarcoma. They are initially small and may be difficult to see, but if growth in size is observed, or when first seen many of them exceed 1 cm in size, the diagnosis is virtually certain.

LINEAR SHADOWS

Linear shadows are common in pneumoconiosis and Kerley has described three types of lines: (A) long linear shadows radiating from the hilum; (B) short horizontal lines in the costophrenic angles; and (C) short curved lines scattered in the lung. All are due to dust in the interlobular septa and possibly also in the lymphatics. Septal lines, particularly the (B) lines, can also be seen in conditions in which there is lymphatic obstruction or distension and in those in which there is interstitial oedema, the septa being engorged with fluid; they thus appear in cardiac failure, particularly due to mitral stenosis or left ventricular failure, and also in neoplasm of the bronchus with hilar glandular lymphatic obstruction. They are also occasionally seen in some stages of pneumonia.

Direct invasion by neoplasm of the radiating lymphatics from the hilum occasionally occurs and gives rise to the condition known as lymphangitis carcinomatosa, with its characteristic linear shadows radiating from the hila*. A similar appearance may be produced by lymphatic obstruction alone and is occasionally seen as a transient feature of acute congestive failure, but the presence of pulmonary oedema, an enlarged heart and distended upper lobe veins in the latter condition should help the distinction to be made.

Longer and thicker horizontal linear shadows in the mid-zones and lower zones are a common sequel to a lung infarct and many of these are now believed to be due to thrombosed pulmonary veins. They have previously been described as Fleischner's lines or linear or plate atelectases.

These linear shadows are different from the fine network or reticular shadowing seen in some forms of sarcoid, rheumatoid lung, scleroderma, other collagen disease, pulmonary fibrosis and a few other rarities; but it is often difficult to distinguish between reticulation and fine nodules. Indeed, it has been shown that the superimposition of many layers of reticulation produces an irregular nodular appearance.

RING SHADOWS

The term ring shadows is used for curved lines forming complete circles, usually air spaces bounded

---

*(A) lines, (B) and (C) lines may also be present from the same cause, and the interlacing lines may produce a reticular or nodular appearance. Enlarged hilar glands are often present, particularly if the neoplasm originates in the abdomen; for example, from the pancreas or the stomach.

by abnormal tissue. Multiple small ring shadows usually basal, but possibly in other segments are seen in bronchiectasis. They also occur in the later stages of many conditions causing widespread fibrosis, such as fibrosing alveolitis, long-standing fibrotic sarcoidosis, rheumatoid disease, histiocytosis X, tuberose sclerosis (honeycomb lung, end-stage lung) and can also be a feature of lymphangitis carcinomatosa. Medium sized ring shadows of varying sizes may be seen in pneumonias with multiple abscesses; for example, staphylococcal or tuberculous bronchopneumonia. Larger sized ring shadows are usually called cavities and are dealt with in the next section.

The foregoing touches very lightly on the subject. The student will find the study of abnormal lung patterns as confusing as it is fascinating, and he must never attempt to make a diagnosis on any single feature of the appearances of the lung fields alone. It must be remembered that the lung may react in a similar way to a large number of disease conditions. It is essential to search the radiograph(s) for other clues to the diagnosis, and although some lung patterns are strongly suggestive of a diagnosis to the experienced observer (experts on industrial disease in particular) it is frequently necessary to rely heavily on clinical and laboratory evidence to arrive at the correct solution.

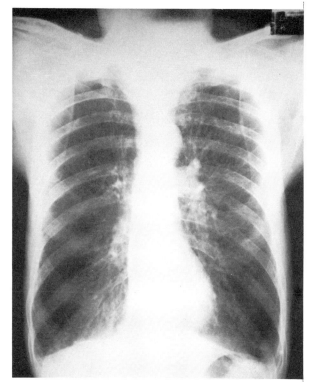

Plate 2.62

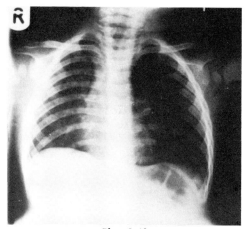

Plate 2.63

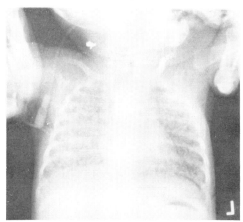

Plate 2.65

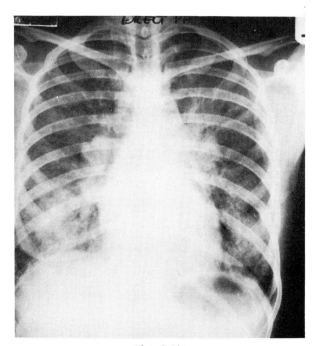

Plate 2.64

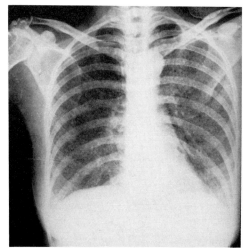

Plate 2.66

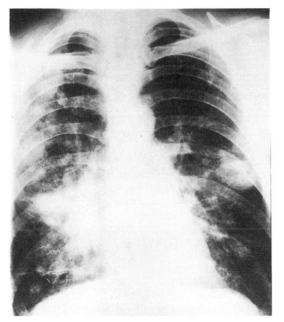

Plate 2.67 (a)

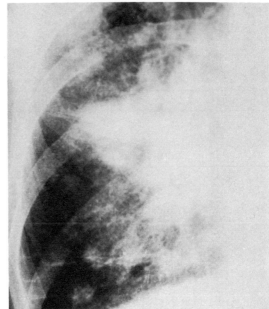

Plate 2.67 (b)

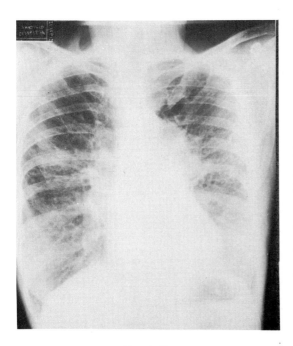

Plate 2.68

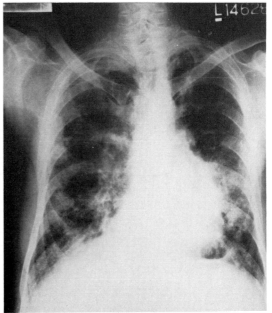

Plate 2.69

SOLUTIONS

Plate 2.62   Expanded rib cage with low flat diaphragms below the anterior end of the 7th rib – almost the 8th – and very poor peripheral lung markings, especially at the bases. The heart is narrow with relative right ventricular enlargement and the proximal hilar vessels are relatively prominent – typical appearances of generalized emphysema.

Plate 2.63   Mediastinum is displaced to the right and the left lung is hypertransradiant; right lung looks normal – typical appearances of 'ball-valve' or obstructive emphysema, due to an inhaled foreign body in the left main bronchus.

Plate 2.64   Bilateral lobulated hilar glandular enlargement with a very fine nodular pattern in the lung fields but blotchy in the lower zones; mixed lung pattern due to sarcoidosis.

Plate 2.65   Infant supported erect. Naso-gastric tube in place. Marked tracheal displacement to right. Widespread miliary shadowing in both lung fields. Miliary tuberculosis, blood spread presumably from massive mediastinal glands.

Plate 2.66   Widespread uniform nodular shadowing. Miliary tuberculosis.

Plate 2.67   (a) and (b) Background fine nodular pattern with basal linear shadows ('A' and 'B' lines) with superimposed larger shadows. Coal-miner's pneumoconiosis with progressive massive fibrosis; detail is shown better in (b).

Plate 2.68   Bilateral hilar lymph gland enlargement, lobulated and asymmetrical, with numerous linear shadows radiating outwards from the hila. Lymphangitis carcinomatosa.

Plate 2.69   Mixed nodular shadowing in mid- and lower zones, predominantly of ring shadows. Widespread bronchiectasis, proved by bronchography.

Abnormal shadows

Broadly speaking, abnormal shadows fall into five groups: (1) large homogeneous shadows (over 1 cm in diameter); (2) irregular shadows of varying density; (3) cavitated shadows; (4) fibrotic shadows; and (5) the 'coin' lesion.

It is, of course, essential to make sure that the shadow in question is really in the lung, since many of the abnormal appearances can be produced by extrapulmonary lesions. Systematic scrutiny should have eliminated many of these possibilities but a lateral view may be needed to confirm this.

LARGE HOMOGENEOUS SHADOW

A large homogeneous shadow should be analysed as follows. Is it:

(1) Compatible with lobar or broncho-pulmonary segmental anatomy? If so it may be pneumonic if consolidated, but segmental or lobar collapse can be produced by bronchial neoplasm in an adult or by a foreign body in a child.

(2) Well-defined, rounded, with sharp edges? If so, then it may be a cyst (bronchial, or hyatid) or a benign lesion (adenoma, chondroma, hamartoma – the two last-named often contain a speck of calcification).

(3) Poorly defined with blurred edges? If so, it is likely to be a neoplasm, although a somewhat similar appearance can be produced by an encysted effusion. Lateral views help in such cases; an encysted effusion shows a lozenge-shaped mass either against the posterior wall of the thorax or in the position of a fissure, and there should also be other evidence of pleural fluid, and of the cause of the effusion, for example, of pulmonary venous hypertension or congestion.

(4) Lobulated? This is very suggestive of neoplasm, particularly if there is a notch or 'hilum' towards the centre of the chest (to receive the abnormal blood vessels).

(5) Waxing and then waning over 3−4 weeks? If not segmental, this would suggest a lung infarct.

In all the foregoing, detail of the lesion may have to be obtained by tomography. It must be stressed that any mass in the lung, whatever its appearance, may be a carcinoma (primary or secondary). Also, any mass which enlarges must be regarded as a carcinoma until proved otherwise.

IRREGULAR SHADOWS OF VARYING DENSITY

These can be extremely confusing. Patches of pulmonary oedema have a fluffy appearance, they may shift in position and tend to disappear under diuretic therapy.

Bronchopneumonia should be included here, although it is more correctly described as confluent nodular shadowing. Pneumonia due to unusual organisms, such as Friedlander's bacillus, or haemophilus, produces large irregular shadows, often in the upper lobes.

Large irregular shadows are seen in the progressive massive fibrosis of coal pneumoconiosis, upper zone or mid-zone, occasionally cavitated, but the diagnosis can usually be made from the associated lung background pattern.

Soft irregular shadows in the upper zones, which may vary in size from 1 cm upwards, are commonly due to tuberculosis. Irregular basal shadows may be produced by an acute reinfection of bronchiectasis, but often there is a lacework background lung pattern in the area involved which permits the diagnosis. A basal shadow which has a streaky horizontal element, and is associated with a small pleural effusion and raised hemidiaphragm is very likely to be due to a lung infarct.

CAVITATED SHADOWS (LARGE RING SHADOWS)

These are most commonly due to tuberculosis (thin walls, sometimes with surrounding involve-ment of lung parenchyma), or to lung abscess (thick walls, smooth interior, normal surrounding lung). Cavitated primary or secondary neoplasm (thick-walled, irregular interior) or broken down hydatid cysts (smooth exterior, irregular contents) do occur. (Rarer causes of thick-walled cavities are Hodgkin's lymphoma, rheumatoid nodule, lung infarct and Wegener's granuloma.) A tuberculous cavity may become secondarily infected with Aspergillus which forms a mycetoma − a ball of fungus lying in the cavity, and slightly smaller than the cavity, so that it is separated from the inner wall by a transradiant crescent of air.

FIBROTIC SHADOWS

The end-result of a number of destructive processes in the lung is fibrosis, as in most inflammatory conditions. This produces lung shrinkage and loss of volume and should first be noted on inspection of the central shadow which may show mediastinal or tracheal shift to the affected side, or of the hila which may be pulled upwards or downwards. The characteristic appearance of localized fibrosis, with numerous parallel or radiating linear shadows of varying thickness often coalescing with dense patches, is easily recognized and is most commonly due to tuberculosis, particularly when associated with pleural thickening and calcifications.

THE 'COIN' LESION

A particular problem is presented by a small, round shadow 0.5−2 cm in diameter with reasonably well-defined edges and no other apparent distinguishing features. If nothing has been gained from studying the remainder of the chest (for example, hilar glands, evidence of secondary deposits or of a primary neoplasm of which this might be a secondary) and the lesion is not cavitated (suggesting tuberculosis or lung abscess, whatever the organism) nor contains calcification (suggesting tuberculoma, hamartoma or chondroma) then it is generally felt essential to regard it as malignant until proved otherwise. It is usually necessary to proceed to tomography in such cases to establish these points of detail.

The foregoing is by no means a complete analysis of the consideration of abnormal lung shadows, and for more detailed description the larger books on chest radiology should be consulted. The intention at this stage is to put forward a basic scheme of approach on which further steps can be built later.

Plates 2.70−2.77 show some typical examples of pleural and lung lesions which should be capable of diagnosis using the information just given.

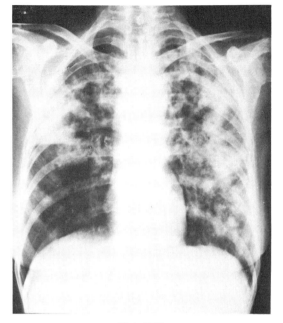

Plate 2.70

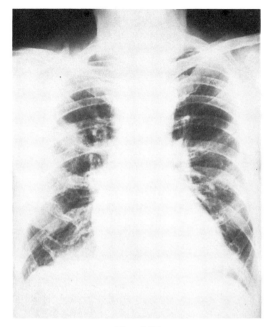

Plate 2.71

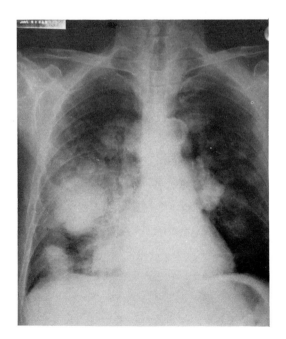

Plate 2.72

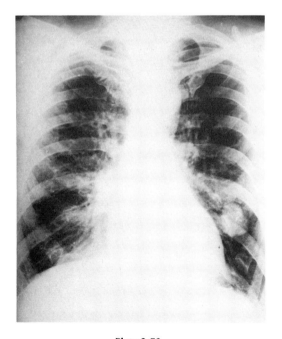

Plate 2.73

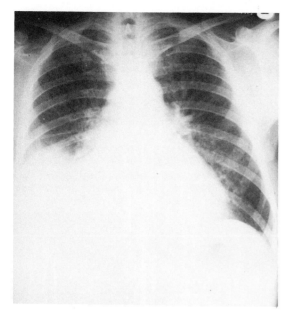

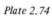

Plate 2.74

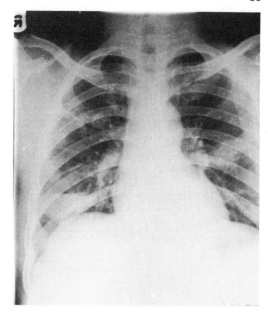

Plate 2.75

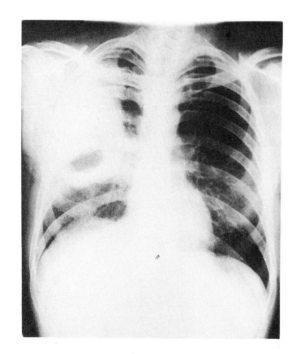

Plate 2.76

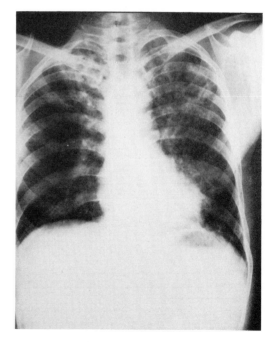

Plate 2.77

SOLUTIONS

Plate 2.70   Widespread patchy shadowing containing numerous ring shadows, rather larger than on Plate 2.69, and sparing the right middle and lower lobe. Might have been a tuberculous bronchopneumonia, but proved to be a staphylococcal pneumonia in a diabetic.

Plate 2.71   Rounded mass in the right upper zone behind the anterior end of the 3rd rib; it has ill-defined edges and seems to be connected to the hilum. This must be presumed to be a neoplasm.

Plate 2.72   Numerous rounded masses of differing sizes throughout the lung fields which must be assumed to be due to secondary deposits.

Plate 2.73   Well-defined mass in the left lower zone; it contains some calcium. This was a hamartoma; the appearance would also have suggested a chondroma.

Plate 2.74   Right diaphragm is raised with horizontal streaky shadowing above it but the horizontal fissure is not displaced. The heart is enlarged due to LV+. ECG monitoring leads in place. Right basal lung infarct.

Plate 2.75   Thin-walled cavity with an air—fluid level in the right lower zone; some old fibrosis in the right upper zone and an ill-defined shadow in the left mid-zone behind the anterior end of the left 3rd rib. This is long-standing tuberculosis showing lesions at three stages. The left mid-zone is the relatively early acute infection, in the right lower zone it has cavitated (this an unusual site, for most tuberculous cavities are seen in the apex of either the upper lobe or the lower lobe) and in the right upper zone a much older lesion has virtually healed leaving only a fibrotic scar. In the absence of the other lesions it would have been much more difficult to have decided about the cause of the cavity.

Plate 2.76   Large thick-walled cavity with considerable surrounding parenchymal involvement of lung tissue, and containing an air—fluid level. Typical appearance of lung abscess. This occurred in a young man; in an older person neoplasm would have to be considered.

Plate 2.77   Extensive irregular soft shadowing in the left upper zone and apex, with a cavity behind the anterior end of the left 2nd rib. There is some ill-defined shadowing in the lower zone with some blurring of the left heart border. This is very likely to be upper lobe tuberculosis, active, with involvement also of the lingula. Less extensive pathology can also be seen in the right apex with a small cavity behind the clavicle.

THE LATERAL VIEW OF THE CHEST

Opinion differs as to the value of the lateral view; in some centres it is hardly ever taken, while in others it is a routine. Nevertheless, it can certainly confirm the presence and location of a lesion in the chest, and help to separate it from normal or abnormal structures and provide additional detail with regard to both shape and internal structure which the PA film may fail to do. Conversely, some information visible in a PA view may be concealed in a lateral view, but the latter is indicated in the following circumstances: (1) unilateral disease (other than apices); (2) abnormalities of the central shadow; and (3) abnormalities of the hila.

The lateral view is of no value in bilateral disease because the two sides are superimposed. In unilateral disease it should be taken with the patient standing erect and with the involved side against the film in order to obtain sharper detail; that side designates it as a right or left lateral view. Not much is lost by taking the wrong lateral view; there is therefore no advantage in taking both lateral views. In central shadow and hilar problems the left lateral view produces less magnification of the heart shadow and is therefore generally preferred. Conventionally, the film is viewed from the 'film' side of the patient, as in the PA film, so that a left lateral view is placed with the sternum to the examiner's left.

Scrutiny of the lateral chest film

The sequence should be similar to that adopted for the PA view, correlating the information from the two films and looking for extra signs.

Soft tissues

Extraneous material and superficial masses should be excluded and the diaphragm studied. Both domes should be visible, with the gastric air-bubble beneath the left. Because of the divergent x-ray beam, the dome of the side nearer the film will be higher and its posterior costophrenic angle against the rib cage not so far back, compared with the side nearer the tube which will show relative magnification (*see Figures 2.13* and *2.14*).

As described earlier in considering the 'outline signs', the diaphragmatic outline will disappear, partially or completely, if there is pleural effusion, basal lung collapse, consolidation or infarct or a mass, solid or cystic, lying against it. The extent of loss is helpful. A large effusion obscures the outline totally and may not be otherwise obvious since it only produces a homogeneous background against the sound lung which looks normal. In front of the oblique fissure, loss of outline indicates right middle lobe or lingular consolidation, and behind it anterior, lateral and posterior basal segmental consolidation or collapse can be identified. True loss of diaphragm occurs in herniation. Hiatus hernia behind the heart shadow, anterior (Morgagni), posterior (Bochdalek), congenital central and traumatic herniae can be identified, but some normal part of the diaphragm is always preserved in a hernia. This distinguishes hernia from eventration or paralysis. In Chilaiditti's syndrome, the gut above and in front of the liver is well shown.

The shoulders, arms, and axillary folds should be noted lest they be mistaken for pathology; they obscure the lung apices, of which the better supplementary view is the tilted apical view.

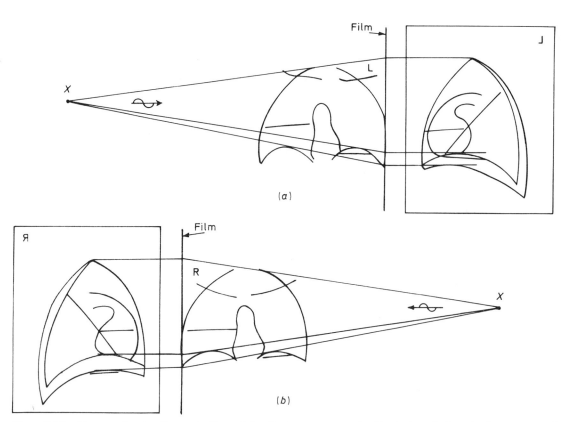

Figure 2.13   Diagram showing the projection of the diaphragms on to the film in lateral view. As the x-rays travel from their point source 'X' they diverge and the image of the diaphragm further from the film is thrown lower than that of the nearer diaphragm, and also is relatively magnified. The effect is more marked on a right lateral film because the right diaphragm is normally higher than the left but is still seen on a left lateral view unless the left diaphragm is abnormally high. The left diaphragm may also be identified by the gastric air-bubble when present, and the diaphragms may also be identified by the fact that the further from the film extends further backwards (see Figure 2.14).

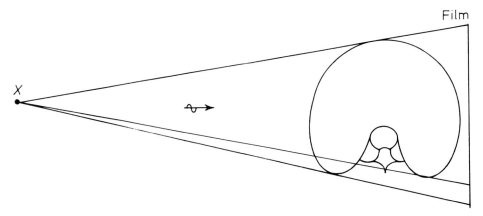

Figure 2.14   Diagram showing how, in a lateral x-ray film of the chest, the posterior parts of the ribs on the side nearer the x-ray tube are projected further back on the film 'f', as the rays diverge from their point source 'X'.

Bony structures

The shoulder girdle and humerus occasionally reveal lesions. The thoracic vertebrae are usually well seen and should be roughly oblong, with a height greater than AP diameter in the upper part, more square lower down, with the anterior border slightly concave and the disc spaces uniform and parallel. In old osteochondritis (Scheuermann's disease) the vertebrae are flattened with narrowed disc spaces and some osteophytosis and small defects in the upper and lower borders (Schmorl's nodes). In early ankylosing spondylitis they look more square, ligamentous ossification occurring later. Disc degeneration with osteophytosis and kyphosis is common in later life. Collapse of a vertebral body may be due to old or recent fracture, infection (tuberculous or staphylococcal usually associated with loss of disc space), neoplasm (usually secondary deposit, occasionally myeloma) or osteoporosis. The latter is a dangerous diagnosis to make on one film alone, even if the classical thinning of the upper and lower cortex of the body is seen throughout the spine, because such bony rarefaction can have other causes, and the appearance may be exaggerated by an over-penetrated or an over-exposed film. Ribs are poorly shown in lateral views due to superimposition, except at the back. Oblique views are better for individual rib lesions. Costal cartilage calcification is evident and the sternum is well shown. The junction between the manubrium and gladiolus, being cartilaginous, is transradiant and should not be mistaken for a fracture. In infants the row of ossific centres will be visible.

The central shadow

The transradiant shadow of the trachea should be followed down from the neck to the carina where it ends in a circular dark shadow due to superimposition of the origin of both main bronchi.

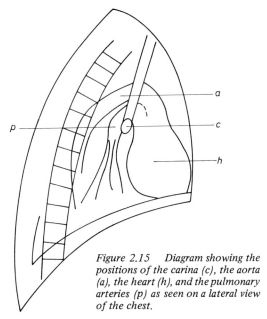

Figure 2.15   Diagram showing the positions of the carina (c), the aorta (a), the heart (h), and the pulmonary arteries (p) as seen on a lateral view of the chest.

From this important landmark other structures can be identified (*Figure 2.15*).

The shadow of the aortic arch can be seen above the carina, curving up in front of, over, and down behind the carina to form the descending aorta which is usually better seen because it overlaps the vertebral bodies. The aortic arch is separated from the carina by the pulmonary arteries but the boundary between these two structures is not radiologically demonstrable where they are in contact because they are of the same radiographic density. They separate out, however, at a point which may lie anywhere from just in front of the level of the carina to just behind it. In front, the aorta is normally separated from the sternum by lung — the two lungs overlie the front of the superior mediastinum and meet somewhere behind the sternum — and this is shown on the film as the 'anterior dark space'. Below this the anterior border of the heart is in contact with the sternum, separated from it by pericardium and retrosternal fat. Since there is usually a thin layer of fat under the visceral pericardium this means that in most lateral films, between the heart and the sternum can be seen two thin transradiant lines on each side of a denser line representing the two layers of the pericardium. If a pericardial effusion is present, the fat layer between the visceral layer of the pericardium will be displaced backwards up to 1.5 cm and may show as a faint transradiancy. This is of some value, since nearly all of the PA appearances which have been described in association with pericardial effusion can be mimicked by other causes of an enlarged heart shadow.

The outline of the heart shadow itself is of less value in determining selective chamber enlargement than in the PA view, but some useful information can be obtained; left ventricular enlargement produces general enlargement backwards but the most prominent part of the curve is towards the lower part, whereas left atrial enlargement tends to produce a well-marked prominence of the middle of the posterior border. An important anatomical landmark, best seen in deep inspiration but not seen in all cases, is the inferior vena cava which can sometimes be noticed passing upwards and forwards from the intercrural diaphragmatic aperture to join the heart shadow from beneath and appreciably in front (though to a variable distance) of the posterior border.

Calcifications should be searched for within the heart shadow. Calcified pericardial plaques are usually much better seen in lateral view than in the PA. Calcified valves (aortic, mitral) may be difficult to distinguish from other overlying calcifications, particularly in the hila, and are much better found by fluoroscopy in the oblique positions.

It is sometimes possible to suggest the diagnosis of superior mediastinal mass from its position in the lateral view. If the anterior dark space is filled in, then the possibilities are, high up, a retrosternal thyroid, an aneurysm of the innominate artery or an oesophageal pouch. A little lower down, glandular enlargement from any cause (inflammatory or neoplastic), thymic tumour or cyst, ectopic thyroid or parathyroid gland, dermoid tumour or cystic hygroma may be the cause. If the mass is in the middle, it may be an aortic aneurysm, enlarged glands, tumour of the oesophagus, bronchogenic cyst, or, again, an ectopic thyroid. Near the diaphragm a rounded shadow with a fluid level presents the typical picture of a hiatus hernia. Posteriorly, a mass is commonly a tumour of neural origin (neurofibroma, ganglioneuroma), but dermoid can also occur; a megaoesophagus due to achalasia of the cardia may be visible the whole way down; paravertebral abscesses or neoplastic deposits may be seen. There are several other, much rarer, causes of such masses and surprises are to be expected.

The hila

Many hilar problems arising in PA films are soluble with the aid of a lateral view. Normally the main pulmonary artery starts in front of the main bronchus and hooks over it, passing above it directed backwards and laterally and then downwards, giving off branches as it does so. It should be seen in front, above and behind the carina, tapering and branching as it goes, although inseparable from the aorta to begin with. Below the carina, only the descending branches are visible (*Figure 2.92*).

Hilar masses which are not vascular in origin do not usually show this pattern; in general, they tend to lie below the level of the carina and may be lobulated or even appear in discrete masses. Even so, it is not always easy to distinguish hilar masses from the vascular pattern, and tomography may be needed. On occasion, what appears to be a hilar mass is shown in lateral view to lie either well behind or well in front of the hilum.

Enlarged pulmonary arteries are usually well shown and are fairly obvious since a substantial part of their bulk lies above and behind the carina, and the branches are traceable.

The lung fields

The normal oblique and horizontal fissures are usually easily seen and should be looked for first.

Some pleural abnormalities are well shown in lateral view — bizarre shadows of pleural calcification, difficult to determine in PA views, may become clarified, and encysted pleural effusions either in the fissures or against the posterior wall are usually easily identified by their position and convexity, and there is often associated alteration of diaphragmatic outline.

Intrapulmonary lesions are often well shown in lateral view except in the apex, and opportunity can be taken to confirm the segmental localization deduced from the PA film. In particular, the relationships with the hila can be determined, and also with the fissures. Discrete lesions not in contact with the central shadow or the diaphragm can only be localized with the aid of a lateral view, and some idea of their nature can be sometimes obtained from the additional view; for example, the lobulated or ill-defined outline of a neoplasm, the presence of calcification in a well-defined lesion as seen in a hamartoma or tuberculoma, a fluid level in a tuberculous cavity or lung abscess, or the so-called 'water-lily' sign in a hydatid cyst. In all these types of lesion, the appearances in lateral views are not vastly different from those to be expected in PA views.

Widespread lesions (nodular or reticular patterns) are not usefully shown on lateral views because of superimposition, although it is sometimes argued that when there is doubt about the presence of nodular shadowing the superimposition of the lung bases will, by exaggerating appearances, make them more obvious.

In summary, lateral views are of great value in confirming, localizing and investigating further many abnormalities seen in PA views.

Some examples will already have been seen in the solutions to the Plates showing PA films, but some further examples are provided in *Plates 2.78–283* which follow.

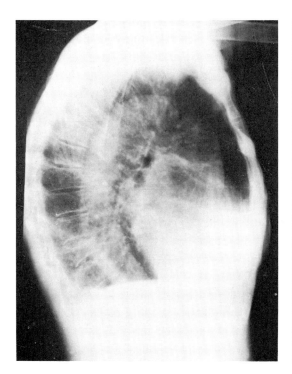

Plate 2.78

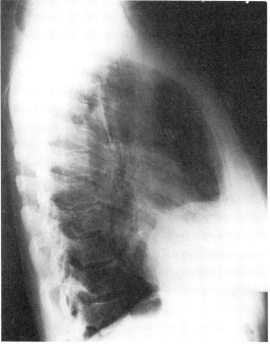

Plate 2.79

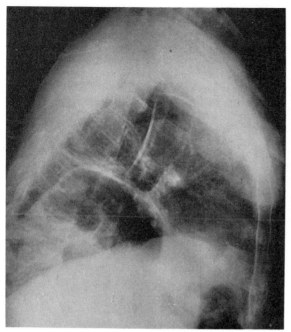

Plate 2.80

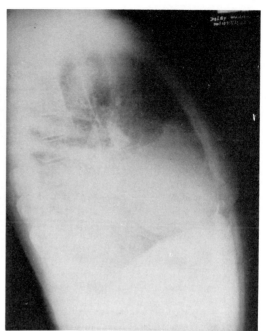

Plate 2.81

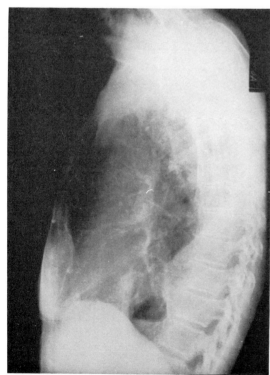

Plate 2.82

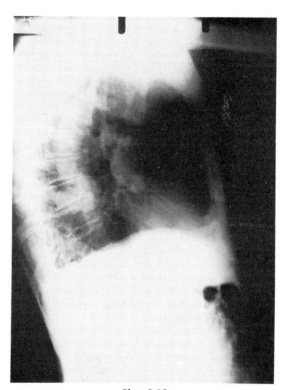

Plate 2.83

SOLUTIONS

Plate 2.78   Anterior wedging of a vertebral body. In this case there was a clear history of recent trauma.

Plate 2.79   Mass in the lower anterior part of the chest with loss of the diaphragmatic outline; it contains some gas shadows. Same case as Plate 2.29; Morgagni hernia. The left diaphragm is identified by the gastric air-bubble beneath it.

Plate 2.80   Only one diaphragmatic outline can be seen complete, and only the anterior part of the other, behind which there is a transradiant region with a well-defined rounded boundary. This is gas-filled gut in a posterior diaphragmatic or Bochdalek hernia on the right. Splenic flexure of colon can be seen above the anterior part of the right and below the left diaphragm.

Plate 2.81   Only one diaphragmatic outline can be seen; the other is masked by the presence of a pleural effusion, the crescentic upper margin of which is easily made out.

Plate 2.82   Only one diaphragmatic outline is seen – the right. The left, identified by the gastric air-bubble beneath it, is obscured by a dense triangular shadow which is due to collapse of the left lower lobe.

Plate 2.83   Lobulated mass in the posterior part of the lower zone, overlying the aorta. This must be regarded as neoplastic until proved otherwise.

CHAPTER 3 | # The Abdomen

Unlike the chest, in which the transradiant air-containing lung provides a dark background contrasting with the denser shadows of normal and pathological structures, the abdomen is composed chiefly of tissues of water density casting relatively dense shadows throughout most of the film. Consequently, organs and tissues are only definable when they are separated by, or contain, air or fat, or overlap to produce double densities.

Transradiancies in the abdomen, often called gas shadows, are most commonly seen in the gut, normal or abnormal, but may also appear in the biliary tree, in abscess cavities, in the peritoneum and, rarely, in air cysts or the portal venous system. The grey shadows due to fat may be seen between the muscle layers of the abdominal wall, beneath the peritoneum and occasionally in fatty tumours.

Where normal organs and tissues of water density are in contact, however, their boundaries are not shown at all. Thus, blood vessels, pancreas, suprarenals, gall bladder, renal collecting systems and ureters, and female organs in the pelvis are virtually invisible. Parts of other organs are also concealed; for example, the upper margin and left lobe of the liver, the upper end of the spleen, and the fluid-filled gut, but the psoas muscle outlines, the lower margin of the liver, the tip of the spleen, the kidneys and sometimes the bladder can usually be made out. Cystic and solid masses may also be similarly concealed, in whole or in part, although if large their increased density and displacement of other structures permit their location.

High density shadows (for example, due to calcification) in organs or tissues may help to identify them, but can also present problems. Bones are usually well seen although detail may be poor in an obese or ascitic abdomen, and in an erect film of the abdomen taken with the patient sitting on the edge of a trolley the pelvis is often concealed.

These unhelpful aspects of plain abdominal radiography have led to the widespread use of radio-opaque contrast media to show the various organs and tissues, the introduction of ultrasound which can show interfaces and distinguish fluid from solid, and the development of computer-assisted tomography which can detect small differences in x-ray absorption.

However, by following an anatomical scheme of scrutiny, and attempting to decide whether the structures visualized are (1) normal (2) abnormal or (3) displaced, much can be learned from a plain film of the abdomen before considering the use of the more sophisticated techniques. The scheme of scrutiny offered here falls conveniently into four groups which further subdivide into four, that is, the boundaries, the bones, the vessels and the organs. The first essential is an appreciation of the radiography.

RADIOGRAPHY

Marking

Correct identification of the patient and of the date on which the film was taken remain essential. Again, the name may suggest the possibility of an exotic disease.

Side

It is even more important in the abdomen to have the left or right side of the patient correctly marked on the film. Situs inversus remains a trap for the unwary, since left-sided biliary colic or acute appendicitis can occur. A normal abdomen is easily 'sided' by the liver in the right upper quadrant, but livers vary in position and can be mimicked on the left by a large spleen, an abscess or a renal or suprarenal tumour. Large masses, cysts, distended gut or defective tissue can displace the liver and other organs.

Position

The erect, supine, prone and lateral decubitus films should be recognized even if they have not been so marked by the radiographer. Erect and supine films are usually taken of an acute abdomen; if the patient is too ill to stand or sit up, the lateral decubitus film may be taken by lying him on one side, usually the left, and by using a horizontal x-ray beam. Supine films are taken in most other conditions, except in pregnancy when the prone position is preferred, thereby reducing radiation to the fetus. The erect film is recognized by the gastric air-bubble with its fluid level, and the air-containing splenic flexure beneath the left diaphragm. Also, in this position, the abdominal organs, especially the fluid-filled gut, droop downwards so that the lower abdomen appears generally more dense. In the lateral decubitus film the gas in the gut or elsewhere floats towards the uppermost side with fluid levels in the long axis of the body. In the supine film the gut gas shadows lie higher up and their anatomy is more easily identified. If the diaphragm is shown there is no gas beneath it since the gastric fundus now contains fluid. If the diaphragm is shown on a prone film, the gastric air-bubble is shown as a crescentic shadow a little way below it, but recognition of the position is easier by noting the apparent increase in width of the sacrum due to the magnification produced by its being nearer to the overcouch x-ray tube when the patient lies back uppermost.

Recognition of these positions will become easier as the student becomes familiar with the appearances to be described in this chapter.

Quality

Correct penetration is essential; the ideal criterion is that the renal outlines be made visible. This is not always possible, but certainly the liver margin should be easily distinguished and the abdominal walls and psoas margins seen.

Respiration

Unlike the chest film, the phase of respiration makes little difference to the appearances of the abdomen but it is essential that the breath be held during exposure of the film (particularly since the exposure times are rather longer in the abdomen), otherwise there will be blurring. All the upper abdominal organs move downwards on inspiration and this movement and certain movements relative to each other can help to distinguish some organs, notably the kidneys and gall bladder.

SCRUTINY OF THE ABDOMEN

Table 3.1

I Boundaries	IV Organs
(1) Diaphragms	(1) Solid organs: liver; spleen;
(2) Abdominal walls	kidneys; suprarenals
(3) Psoas muscles	(2) Hollow organs: renal
(4) Peritoneum	collecting system and
	ureter; stomach; biliary
II Bones	system (gall bladder, biliary
(1) Lower ribs	tree, pancreatic duct, pan-
(2) Costal cartilages	creas); intestine (duodenum,
(3) Lumbar spine	jejunum, ileum, colon)
(4) Pelvis	(3) Pelvic organs: sigmoid
	colon; rectum; bladder;
III Vessels	female organs or male organs
(1) Arteries	(4) Abnormal and unanatomical
(2) Veins	shadows: gas shadows;
(3) Lymphatics	fat shadows; water density
(4) Lymph glands	shadows; high density
	shadows

BOUNDARIES
(*see Figure 3.1*)

Diaphragms

Start by inspecting the diaphragms: in a supine film of the abdomen they may not be included but should always be shown in an erect film. The right diaphragm is normally higher than the left, continuous with the liver shadow below and medially often continuous with the heart shadow above. On the left, the diaphragm is usually visible through the heart shadow, and beneath it from right to left are the left lobe of liver, the gastric fundus, the spleen and often the splenic flexure of the colon, the position of which is variable. In an erect film the fundus contains the gastric air-bubble but in the supine position it contains gastric juice and so may be indistinguishable or, occasionally, represented by a round

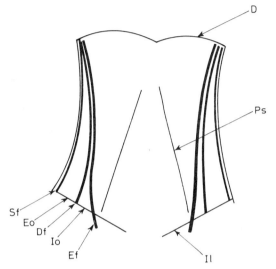

Figure 3.1 Diagram showing the radiological boundaries of the abdomen. D–diaphragm; Sf–superficial fascia; EO–external oblique muscle; Df–deep fascia; Io–internal oblique muscle; Ef–extraperitoneal fat ('flank stripe'); Ps–psoas muscle margin; Il–Inguinal ligament.

shadow of slightly increased density. An absent gastric air-bubble in the erect position should lead to careful scrutiny of the central shadow in the chest film since it is often associated with either a hiatus hernia or achalasia of the cardia (*see* Chapter 2), but it can be displaced by a mass. If one diaphragm is not visible, there may be an effusion or collapsed lung above it. (A pneumonia or lung infarct occasionally simulates an acute abdomen clinically.) Additional gas shadows beneath the diaphragms may be of three types: (1) in hollow organs; (2) free in the peritoneum; or (3) in abscess cavities.

Occasionally, the colon lies between the anterior abdominal wall and the liver and it separates the liver from the anterior part of the diaphragm — Chilaiditti's syndrome — on the right. In acute intestinal obstruction, gas-filled loops of dilated small gut are sometimes seen beneath the left diaphragm. Free gas in the peritoneum is usually seen as a thin, crescentic, dark shadow separating the liver from the diaphragm on the right and the

stomach and splenic flexure from it on the left, usually, though not always, on both sides simultaneously. It may be more extensive with downward displacement of organs. Linear fat shadows should not cause confusion but a stomach containing food residues or blood clot may produce a roughly crescentic gastric air-bubble.

Gas in a subphrenic abscess is usually unilateral and more circumscribed, with a horizontal fluid level below the gas, and should be separable from the gastric air-bubble and splenic flexure on the left. There is often an associated small pleural effusion above it. On the right, gas in a liver abscess may look somewhat the same, but will tend to lie slightly lower.

Abdominal walls

The lateral abdominal walls, from without inwards, should show skin, a layer of fat, external oblique muscle, another thin layer of fat, internal oblique muscle and then a thicker layer of extraperitoneal fat extending from the costal margin down to the iliac fossa — sometimes known as the 'flank stripe'. Part of these fat layers may disappear if the region is involved in an inflammatory lesion such as an extensive perinephric abscess, a pericolic abscess or sometimes an appendix abscess. The hernial orifices should be noted at this stage, remembering that the inguinal ligament runs from the anterior superior iliac spine to the pubic tubercle and no gut shadows should normally be visible below this line. Ventral or incisional hernias sometimes produce confusing shadows, and in the large pendulous abdomen, skin folds often produce a relatively dense shadow, curved convex downwards across the film.

Note should also be taken of the gluteal muscles, which sometimes contain evidence of previous intramuscular injections in the form of rounded or streaky opacities. If very dense they may be due to bismuth preparations formerly used in the treatment of syphilis.

Psoas outlines

The psoas outlines are not well seen on every film but can be made out in most. They are roughly symmetrical, starting at the upper angles of L1, crossing the transverse processes of that vertebra and widening out as they run downwards to disappear into the pelvis just lateral to the sacro-iliac joints. The outline may be lost in retroperitoneal lesions such as haematoma, urinary extravasation, abscess or tumour, and they may be displaced laterally by a paravertebral abscess (usually tuberculous) or a similarly placed mass.

Peritoneum

The peritoneum should be reconsidered at this stage. Normally invisible, it may be outlined by free gas beneath the diaphragm in the erect film or between the lateral wall and the abdominal organs in the lateral decubitus view. In the supine position the gas will form a thin layer beneath the anterior abdominal wall and will not be visible on an AP view, although a lateral view with a horizontal x-ray beam may show it.

Free gas in the peritoneum may occur in perforated peptic ulcer, perforated intestinal ulcer or neoplasm, penetrating wounds, ruptured gut after blunt injury, after abdominal operations or peritoneal dialysis and in diagnostic or therapeutic pneumoperitoneum including tubal insufflation.

If the peritoneum contains a lot of fluid (ascites) the film generally looks much more dense than usual and detail is difficult to make out, due to excessive scatter of the radiation, with a generally light grey look. If coils of gut are shown by the gas they contain they are in the middle of the abdomen, further apart than usual in supine view, rising into the upper abdomen in erect view. This is different from the centrifugal distribution of gut round a large ovarian cyst (*see* page 91). In the supine lateral view, with a horizontal beam, the gut may be seen floating on top of the fluid.

Now study *Plates 3.1–3.4,* each of which shows an abnormality of the boundaries.

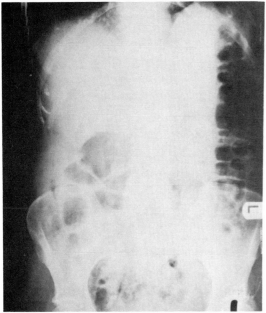
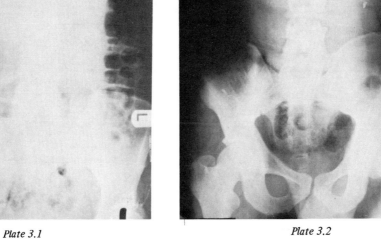

Plate 3.1

Plate 3.2

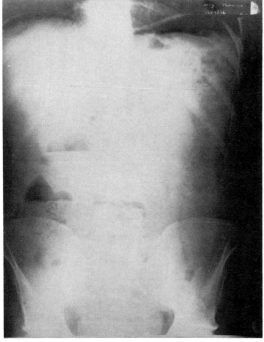
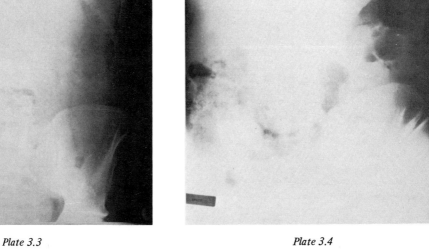

Plate 3.3

Plate 3.4

SOLUTIONS

Plate 3.1   Normal shadow of the abdominal wall cannot be seen on the right. The lateral wall is oedematous with a longitudinal gas shadow. This was a pericolic abscess pointing in the right loin.

Plate 3.2   Note loss of right psoas margin. Severe injury due to road traffic accident, with large retroperitoneal haematoma.

Plate 3.3   Erect film of the abdomen. Free gas in the peritoneal cavity, seen here between the liver and the diaphragm on the right and between the diaphragm and the stomach on the left, distinguishable from the gastric air-bubble, although the wall of the gastric fundus is a little difficult to see. The dome of the left diaphragm is obscured by the name—date marker.

Plate 3.4   Erect film of the abdomen, showing a large collection of gas beneath the diaphragm on each side. A fluid level can be seen on the right. On the left, the lower part of the subdiaphragmatic gas shadow is outlined by a curvilinear structure ending laterally in a short linear opacity. This is a gastric tube with an opaque tip, confirming that the left-hand collection of gas is in the stomach, so that the unilateral collection of gas on the right is most likely to be in a subphrenic abscess.

THE BONES

The lower ribs

The 10th, 11th and 12th ribs are usually well demonstrated. The 12th rib usually overlies the kidney and some part of it will have to be excised for kidney surgery. Rib fractures may occur in road traffic accidents and other injuries and occasionally secondary deposits of neoplasm or myeloma, or infective processes (for example, tuberculosis) may be an unsuspected cause of pain in the renal area.

The costal cartilages

Although often invisible, the costal cartilages can be calcified and those of the 6th to 10th ribs are often shown in the upper part of a film of the abdomen. If the calcification is extensive, there is no difficulty in identification from the pattern of parallel lines curved convex downwards and then sloping upwards to the xiphisternum. The difficulty arises when there are only odd spots of calcification and they may overlie the liver, or gall bladder on the right and the left lobe of the liver or spleen on the left of the kidney or suprarenal on both sides.

Problems are usually readily solved by taking a lateral view of the upper abdomen when costal cartilage calcification will be seen to lie in the anterior wall of the trunk; on the right, an oblique view of the gall bladder area may be used. On inspiration, the costal cartilages usually move upwards in relation to upper abdominal organs, while the gall bladder moves downwards and outwards. The point here is that there is no difficulty in preventing confusion caused by costal cartilage calcifications providing they are remembered and considered at an early stage of scrutiny of the film.

The lumbar spine

Inspection of the lumbar spine should be done up and down four times, first, to look at the vertebral bodies, then the transverse processes, followed by the pedicles and, finally, the laminae and spinous processes. Congenital variations such as fusion, hemivertebra and unusual somatic segmentation may occur; for example, there may be four or six lumbar vertebrae, the lowest lumbar or upper sacral vertebra being transitional in type with large or asymmetrical transverse processes. Partial or complete collapse of a vertebral body may be due to a compression fracture, infection (tuberculous or staphylococcal are commonest) or neoplasm, usually secondary − there are other rarer causes. Multiple collapse can occur in osteoporosis and also in myelomatosis. Bony defects are commonly due to secondary neoplasm (for example, a missing pedicle or spinous process). Increased density of a single vertebral body can be due to Paget's disease (when it is usually slightly enlarged with coarse trabeculation), secondary neoplasm or Hodgkin's disease, and multiple osteolytic or osteosclerotic (or mixed) secondary deposits may occur. Erosion of several vertebrae from the left may be due to aortic aneurysm. Involvement of spinal nerves in vertebral disease can produce pain mimicking that from any abdominal organ.

Pelvis

In the pelvis, more obvious abnormalities such as hip disease or old fractures may be noted. Deformities due to bone softening as in osteomalacia or

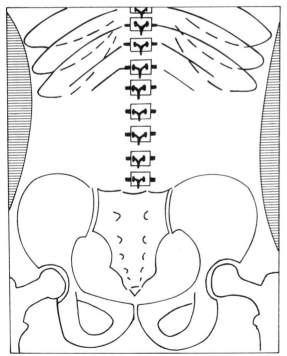

Figure 3.2   Diagram showing the bony structures − ribs, costal cartlages, spine and pelvis − which may be visible on a plain film of the abdomen.

rickets may be seen and alterations in bone texture or trabeculation should be noted. Increased density with a thickened cortex usually indicates Paget's disease, and osteosclerotic or osteolytic lesions of metastatic neoplasms should be looked for; the latter rarely alter the size and shape of a bone unless there is a pathological fracture. Larger bone defects due to destructive neoplasm may easily be confused with gut shadows; if in doubt, the cortex should be traced carefully round the various bones of the pelvis and then the bone trabeculations compared on the two sides.

Now study *Plates 3.5–3.8* and look for bony lesions in the abdomen.

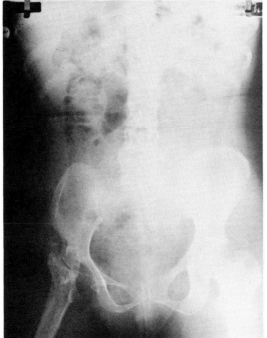
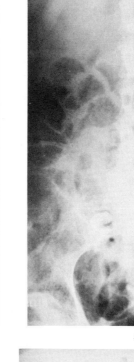

Plate 3.5

Plate 3.6

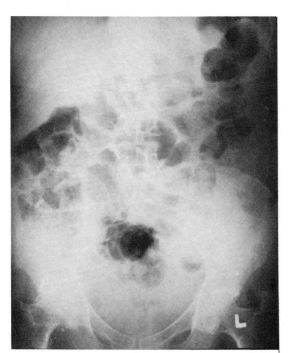
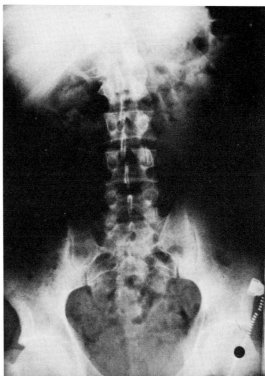

Plate 3.7

Plate 3.8

SOLUTIONS

Plate 3.5   The body of L4 is compressed with extruded lateral fragments, due to previous trauma. The head and neck of the right femur are absent, and the remaining upper end of the femur appears to have fractured following arthrodesis and has formed a false joint with the acetabular roof. This is a long-standing condition, since the right half of the pelvis is underdeveloped, and must date from late childhood.

Plate 3.6   There is a defect in the medial part of the right ilium; on the left, the upper cortex of the iliac crest can be traced downwards and medially past the transverse process of L5 into the sacro-iliac joint, but on the right there is a gap. This was due to a secondary deposit from a urothelial tumour. Note also the increased density of the body of L5, in this case due to osteo-arthritis, and a dense shadow overlying L3, L4 and L5 due to oily contrast medium retained in the spinal theca from a previous myelogram.

Plate 3.7   The right hip joint shows increased density and a narrowed joint space, barely visible on this film. It is just possible to see small osteophytes at the edge of the joint. This is osteoarthritis of the right hip.

Plate 3.8   Thoraco-lumbar scoliosis concave to the right, which is compensating for a congenital anomaly of the lower thoracic region. The left 11th rib and the right half of the body of T11 is absent, and the 10th and 12th left ribs are fused. Note also trouser zip-fastener over the left hip joint, and a small dark round shadow due to a serial number marker.

VESSELS

All the blood and lymph vessels are indistinguishable in the abdomen except in certain circumstances.

Arteries

Calcification associated with atheroma or arteriosclerosis of various kinds can occur in the aorta, the splenic artery and the iliac arteries; it is much less common in other vessels. Aneurysmal dilatation of the aorta (usually arteriosclerotic) may be seen as a soft-tissue mass commonly on the left side of the lumbar spine and it often has a calcified rim. It is also visible in the lateral view; on rare occasions, a large long-standing aneurysm will provide erosion of vertebral bodies, presumably due to the increased pulsation against them.

Arteries will, of course, be seen if opacified at arteriography by the injection of contrast medium.

Veins

Again, veins are normally indistinguishable, being of water density, but in the pelvic venous plexus phleboliths are common causes of small rounded opacities varying from 2–5 mm in size; they are of no clinical significance except that they may look just like lower ureteric stones. The iliac veins and inferior vena cava may be opacified at venography. Rarely, in portal pyaemia (and necrotizing entero-colitis — *see* page 82), gas may appear in veins in the liver.

Lymphatics

Normally invisible, the lymphatics may be demon-strated by lymphography. The oily contrast medium may persist in them for some time and the charac-teristic appearance and location of these fine linear opacities should be easily recognized. The procedure is usually associated with the investi-gation or management of some form of malignant disease, or with some type of pathology of the lymph pathways in the legs.

Lymph glands

Large gland masses are occasionally visible in the para-aortic chain, but the commonest appearance is of old calcified mesenteric glands (due pre-sumably to defeated old tuberculous infection) seen almost anywhere in the area occupied by the gut but usually along the line of posterior attach-ment of the mesentery. They are mobile, seen in different places on supine, erect and other films and have a characteristic irregular spotty and craggy appearance. They are of no clinical sig-nificance but must be correctly recognized to prevent their being mistaken for anything else. Occasionally, of course, they are atypical in appearance when differentiation may be difficult, but demonstration of their location and mobility is usually enough.

Vessels are visible in *Plates 3.9* and *3.10*.

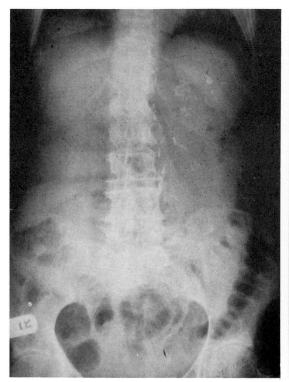
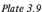

Plate 3.9

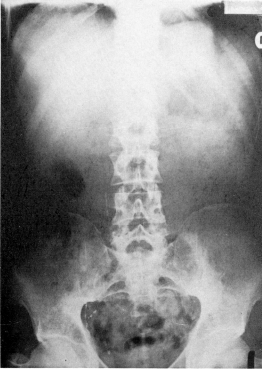

Plate 3.10

SOLUTIONS

Plate 3.9 Irregular calcification in the upper left quadrant of the abdomen is in the splenic artery. There is a rounded mass to the left of the spine with a rim of calcification round its lateral margin and some linear streaks of calcification down its medial border — this is the typical appearance of an aortic aneurysm.

Plate 3.10 Linear dense shadows to the right of the spine and in the lateral part of the pelvis are due to contrast medium in the lymphatics following lymphography.

ORGANS

Solid organs

LIVER

The most obvious organ is the liver, producing a dense triangular shadow in the right hypochondrium with its lower edge running obliquely close to the costal margin. While many differing shapes may be seen, most livers have a long horizontal axis, the lateral part of the lower margin being just above the costal margin and the remainder of the lower border extending upwards and medially to cross the midline just below the xiphisternum, where the left lobe begins. It seems to 'tail' off here. In a small but appreciable proportion of cases, particularly in women, the liver lies entirely on the right of the midline, with the long axis vertical, a substantial part of the right lobe lying below the costal margin. If the ribs indent the liver on its lateral side, usually in women, that portion below is sometimes called a Reidl's lobe.

The upper surface of the liver is normally applied closely to and indistinguishable from the right diaphragm unless separated from it by free intraperitoneal gas, or gas in the colon above and in front, (as described above and in Chapter 2). Any other transradiant gas shadows in the liver area may be either in a subphrenic abscess (whose boundaries with the diaphragm and the liver will not be indistinguishable, all being of water density) or in a liver abscess itself. Differentiation between these two conditions may be difficult, even with

films in different positions, or with fluoroscopy. The most useful is an AP film in the lateral decubitus position, right side up, when the lateral limit of the gas shadow can be seen. Gas may also be seen in hepatic veins or the biliary tree.

The liver may be actually enlarged if it contains an abscess (non-specific or amoebic) or a tumour (primary, hepatoma, or secondary, commonly from gut, but any other tumour may metastasize to the liver) and apparently enlarged in the presence of right subphrenic abscess which displaces it downwards. In the absence of gas shadows in the abscess, or of associated basal lung reaction or effusion, plain radiography will not distinguish between these causes of lowering of the lower edge of the liver (radioisotope scanning and ultrasound 'B' scan may be of more help).

Calcification within the liver may occur in a number of conditions, notably cysts of congenital origin, old injuries, old abscesses, hydatid cysts, old infarcts, neoplasms (more commonly hepatoma, especially in children) and, rarely, syphilitic gummata. Stones occasionally ascend the biliary tree.

SPLEEN

The spleen is often difficult to see on a straight film although its tip can often be made out inside the rib cage. In the supine position, the upper or medial pole is not seen because it is related directly to the fundus of the stomach which usually contains some gastric juice, and these shadows of water density are, of course, indistinguishable. A special projection, with the patient prone and the right side raised 10 degrees, is of value to show the whole outline; this is because the gastric fundus contains some air in the prone position — *see* page 64.

An enlarged spleen is readily visible and the same rule applies as in clinical medicine; that is to say, if the tip is below the costal margin the spleen is three times its normal size. If very large the borders of the spleen may not be so obvious and the only effect is an extensive diffuse shadow over the whole of the left side of the abdomen; it may be necessary, therefore, as in physical examination, to search for the tip in the right iliac fossa. Calcification in the spleen is uncommon, but if present may be due to a cyst, an old injury or infarct, old tuberculosis, abscess or hydatid cyst; phleboliths may also occur.

KIDNEYS

The kidneys should nearly always be seen in a plain film of the abdomen. However, the renal outline is only visible on account of the perinephric fat and where this is lacking difficulties will be found. If there is a good deal of gas or faecal matter in the gut, which conceals this, or the patient is thin, ill and/or aged, or the film is incorrectly exposed, they may not be visible. In fat people they are usually well shown. Much will depend on the skill of the radiographer.

Normally, the kidneys overlie the 12th rib on both sides, the upper poles tilted slightly medially and the right kidney normally lying 1 or 2 cm below the left (apparently displaced downwards by the liver), but this asymmetry in height is very variable and may even be reversed without significance. The right kidney may descend almost into the right iliac fossa or be tucked up behind the liver and still be normal. If the tilt is lost or reversed and the lower poles are not traceable, horse-shoe kidney may be suspected. Changes in the size of the kidneys are of considerable importance — a difference of over 1.5 cm in length is significant. The normal range is from 10 to 15 cm in the adult (more commonly 11—14 cm) but the length is related to age in children and to body surface area in adults; there is also a reasonable relationship with height. (A useful set of graphs showing the relationship to age and height has been published by Kodak from data assembled by Hodson *et al.,* 1962.) An attempt should also be made to determine whether the outline is smooth or irregular or whether any 'lumps' are present. Such observations are, however, not usually easy to make with certainty on a plain film (although they can often be suspected), and if there is reasonable suspicion of renal disease it is usual to proceed to intravenous urography.

There are several reasons why one renal outline may not be seen when the other is visible. The kidney may not be there at all; it may be congenitally absent or have been removed surgically (part of the 12th rib — sometimes the 11th rib also — will probably have been removed during the surgical approach in such a case), or it may be somewhere else; that is, ectopic, usually in the pelvis. The outline may be blurred, in whole or in part, usually due to fluid infiltrating the capsule and abolishing the transradiant effect of the perinephric fat, for example, haemorrhage following trauma, urine following pelvic or calycine rupture due to trauma or to back pressure (rare) or pus as in some types of perinephric abscess. More commonly only part of the outline is blurred. Movement of the kidney during respiration will, of course, produce the well known radiographic effect of respiratory blur and, conversely, haemorrhage or pain may inhibit such movement and prevent this effect. Finally, the kidney may be so large that the outlines are concealed against the boundaries of the abdomen, and the medial border may be masked over the spine or may project well beyond it. Such an effect is usually due to obstructive disease, commonly pelvi-ureteric junction obstruction, but a very large tumour or cyst may be the cause, especially in children.

Opacities in the renal area are always of interest and should be studied closely. If they occur in the kidney they may be either in the renal substance or in the collecting system. In the latter case, they are most likely to be stones, although a papilloma of the renal pelvis occasionally calcifies, and calcification is a marked feature of old tuberculous pyonephrosis. If the collecting system or a calyx containing a stone is greatly dilated it will be difficult, without intravenous urography, to be sure exactly where the opacity is.

There is a relatively long list of causes of opacities in the renal substance, but they may be broadly grouped into localized calcifying lesions and more widespread and scattered small calcifications more usually called nephrocalcinosis. The former may be due to congenital or other cysts, old injuries, old tuberculous infections, old infarcts, renal carcinoma or other tumours.

Nephrocalcinosis occurs in several chronic hypercalcaemic conditions, notably hyperparathyroidism, widespread secondary osteolytic neoplastic deposits, myelomatosis and generalized sarcoidosis and in renal tubular acidosis. The appearance is of short radial dense streaks at the sites of the cortico-medullary junctions at the bases of the renal pyramids. In another condition, medullary sponge kidney, small stones may form in the tiny cysts in the medulla adjacent to the calyces, and these tend to lie nearer the hilum of the kidney than the opacities of true nephrocalcinosis. The differentiation can be difficult on a plain film and intravenous urography will be needed to locate the calcifications with respect to the calyces.

What matters in the scrutiny of a plain film of the abdomen, however, is not so much the need to arrive at a definitive diagnosis of an opacity in the renal area as the need to prove that it lies within the kidney or the collecting system, so indicating the necessity to proceed to intravenous urography. Such proof is usually obtained either by taking films in both inspiration and expiration, by taking an oblique view, or by studying erect and supine films. An intrarenal opacity will remain in fixed relationship to the renal outline wherever that may be.

SUPRARENALS

Occasionally, the suprarenals are visible on top of the upper poles of the kidneys but more usually they are not shown; a large tumour in the suprarenal gland may be visible as a mass above the kidney. On the left it is important not to mistake the fluid-filled fundus of the stomach, which may look almost circular in the supine position, for such a tumour (this false appearance will disappear on a prone film). Calcification in the suprarenal glands occurs in old tuberculous infection, usually bilateral, which is associated with Addison's disease (the combination of weakness, diarrhoea and skin pigmentation with suprarenal calcification is diagnostic), and also in neuroblastoma arising from the gland (usually unilateral, and in a child). Smaller tumours of this region such as phaeochromocytoma or the adenoma or hyperplasia of Cushing's syndrome require special techniques for their demonstration (for example, arteriography, venography, retroperitoneal air insufflation).

Now study *Plates 3.11–3.15* which show abnormalities of solid organs.

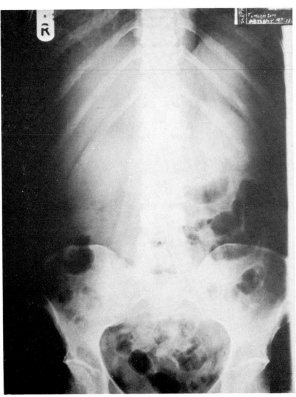

Plate 3.11

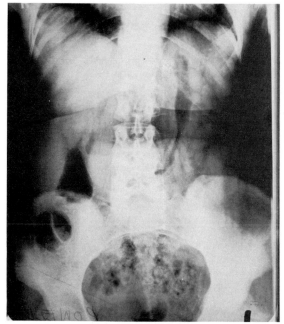

Plate 3.12

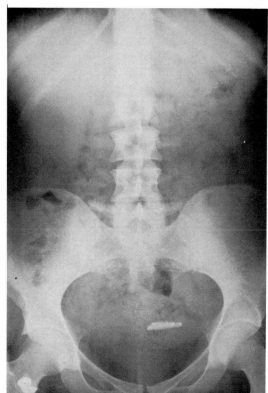

Plate 3.13

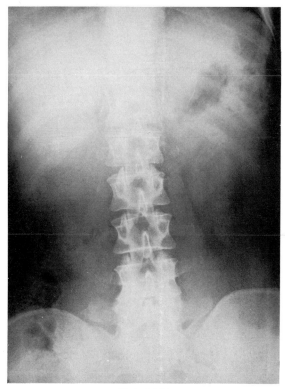

Plate 3.14

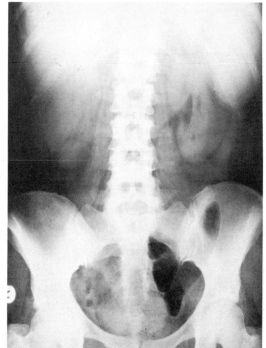

Plate 3.15

SOLUTIONS

Plate 3.11   Increased shadowing in the upper part of the abdomen is due to enlargement of the liver. The gastric air-bubble in the pyloric antrum and the gas in the transverse colon and the splenic flexure are displaced downwards. Cirrhosis of the liver was the cause in this case though, of course, this cannot be diagnosed from the film.

Plate 3.12   Calcifications on each side of the lower thoracic spine can be seen to be just above the upper poles of the kidneys and are in the suprarenal glands – a patient with Addison's disease.

Plate 3.13   Right renal outline is well seen but the left is difficult to make out. The distal part of the left 11th rib is missing. The left kidney has been removed on account of tuberculous infection. Note also intra-uterine contraceptive device in the pelvis (Lippe's loop). Absence of the left kidney is confirmed on intravenous urography (Plate 3.16).

Plate 3.14   Normal left renal outline can just be made out, particularly its lower pole, but on the right, below the liver margin, there is a large soft-tissue mass containing some calcification, below which the remainder of a normal renal outline can be seen but displaced downwards. This could be a suprarenal or renal tumour, the type of calcification rather suggesting the latter. It was shown to be a renal carcinoma.

Plate 3.15   The spleen is enlarged. There is some enlargement of the liver also but it is not obvious on this film.

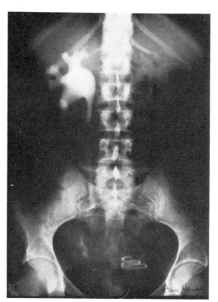

Plate 3.16

Hollow organs

RENAL COLLECTING SYSTEM AND URETERS

These are normally invisible on a plain film but an enlarged renal pelvis due to pelvi-ureteric junction obstruction is occasionally outlined. Reference has already been made to a kidney and renal pelvis so large as to 'disappear'. Stones in the renal pelvis show as opacities lying medial to the kidney but they may not be in constant relationship to it nor to the lumbar spine if mobile within the renal pelvis, and again intravenous urography will be needed to prove the relationship. Stones in the ureter should lie along its anticipated line which in most cases is along the tips of the transverse processes, but tending to be more lateral lower down, and curving out laterally in the pelvis to swing in medially towards the bladder base. Ureteric stones may be of any size from 2 mm to 2 cm, but 4—5 mm in diameter is common. It should be added that it may be very difficult to see a small ureteric stone if it overlies bone, either over a transverse process or over the sacral ala; consequently, if a stone should move up or down the ureter or even change position because of a different phase of respiration at the moment the film is taken, it may 'disappear' over bone, to reappear on a subsequent film.

STOMACH

The stomach is no more than a shaped tube of muscle, containing a variable amount of fluid and gas; being thus mostly of water density. It is inseparable radiologically from other organs and is only identifiable on plain films by its gas-bubble, which shows as a transradiancy or dark area. It is worth looking at films of the normal barium-filled stomach to get a general idea of its shape in life as shown diagrammatically in *Figure 3.3*. It is important to appreciate that the fundus lies beneath the left diaphragm *behind* the coronal plane in the left paravertebral gutter, and that the pyloric antrum lies in front of the spine and therefore *in front* of the coronal plane. It follows that in the erect position the gastric air-bubble is in the fundus beneath the left diaphragm (the rest of the stomach not being visualized), while in the supine position it moves to what is then the highest point of the stomach from the ground, the pyloric antrum in front of the spine. There is some variability in the position of the antrum about the midline and consequently the shape of the gastric air-bubble in the supine position is likewise somewhat variable. On occasions, gastric rugae can be made out which helps to identify it. It should always be above and parallel to the gas shadows of the transverse colon, to which it is loosely joined by the greater omentum. A large pancreatic cyst may separate these two structures, and other masses may displace the stomach. An enlarged liver may displace it downwards and to the left, and a large spleen may displace it to the right.

It is not usual to obtain much detailed information about intragastric lesions from a plain film, but in a severe pyloric stenosis from either pyloric or duodenal ulcer, or involvement in malignant disease, the stomach may contain a lot of fluid and food residues, and its gas-bubble will

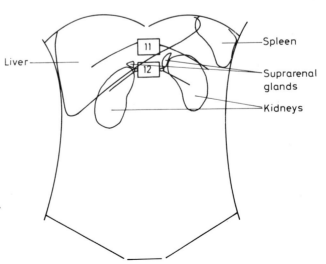

Figure 3.3 Diagram showing the common position of the solid organs in a supine film of the abdomen. Note that the right kidney usually lies lower than the left, and that both are related to the 12th rib, and sometimes to the 11th rib.

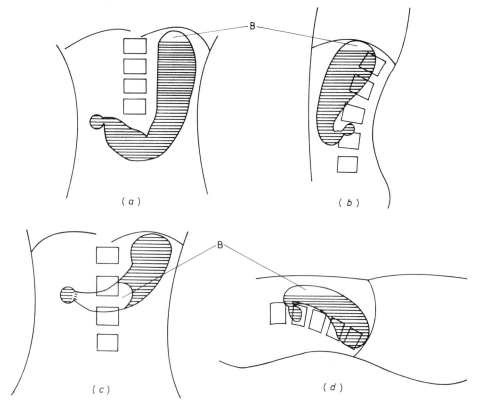

Figure 3.4   Diagrams showing the different positions of the gastric air-bubble (B) in the erect and supine positions. It clearly rises to the highest point. (a) AP erect. (b) Erect lateral. (c) AP supine. (d) Supine lateral.

be larger. There is sometimes a second bubble in the pyloric antrum. The transverse colon will be displaced downwards. If the food residues include much solid matter, the same coarsely speckled appearance is seen as occurs in the dilated oesophagus of achalasia or in faecal matter in the colon. Indeed, it may need very careful scrutiny to distinguish such a stomach from splenic flexure of the colon.

BILIARY SYSTEM

The *gall bladder* is not usually visible, being of water density. Occasionally, in obstructive conditions such as neoplasm involving the cystic duct, there is a good deal of calcium in the stagnant bile and the gall bladder becomes opaque — so-called 'limey bile'. Usually the only visible indication of gall bladder disease is the presence of opaque stones which may be of variable size — the larger the more likely are they to be faceted and laminated — concentric layers of calcified material producing a characteristic appearance. However, the type of calcification is variable and sometimes it appears homogeneous or spiculated. It is important to remember that a large proportion of gall stones are only pigmented and are not calcified. They are, in supine view, usually located just below the costal margin and the inferior edge of the liver just above the hepatic flexure of colon and lateral to the duodenal cap. They are distinguished from renal stones by their movement downwards and inwards on inspiration and by their anterior position shown on a lateral or oblique view. Widely separated or mobile gall stones suggest a distended gall bladder full of fluid.

Occasionally, if there is air in the biliary tree it may enter the gall bladder, but this is unusual; if the gall bladder is infected with gas-forming organisms the wall may be infiltrated with gas which may be visible as dark shadows outlining the organ.

The *biliary tree* is normally invisible on a plain film. It can contain gas and so be shown as a dark transradiancy after biliary surgery involving by-pass to the gut (for example, in cholecystenterostomy or choledochenterostomy) or in the condition known as 'gall-stone ileus' in which a large gall stone ulcerates through the fundus of the gall bladder into the neighbouring duodenum, passes down the gut and eventually obstructs it. The combination of gas in the biliary tree from the fistula with the duodenum, dilated small gut due to the obstruction and an opacity low in the abdomen is diagnostic. Occasionally, dense shadows of obstructed gut full of fluid may obscure the stone, or it may be non-opaque.

Stones in the biliary tree, as a cause of obstructive jaundice, may be calcified and visible lying to the right of the upper lumbar and may have to be distinguished from renal stones, calcified lymph glands or calcification in suprarenal gland.

The *pancreatic duct* is not normally visible though it may contain calculi.

The *pancreas* is radiologically invisible and remains the abdominal organ most inaccessible to investigative techniques. If calcified (as in chronic pancreatitis) a collection of dots running across the abdomen from the spine upwards into the left hypochondrium gives away its position but pancreatic tumours cannot be seen unless they are so large as to displace or deform other more visible organs. A cyst or large tumour of the head of the pancreas will enlarge the duodenal loop and elevate the pyloric antrum while displacing the transverse colon downwards, and a large cyst of the body may displace the stomach to the right and the transverse colon downwards. A large cyst of the head may also extend upwards and displace the stomach downwards and to the left.

INTESTINE

The *duodenum* is not usually visible on a plain film but gas can sometimes be seen in the duodenal cap or bulb (at the beginning of the first part). This is more likely to occur if there is any obstruction to movement through the duodenum, such as ulcer at the apex of the cap or a post-bulbar ulcer, a duodenal diaphragm, obstruction of the fourth part of the duodenum by malrotation or tumour of the pancreas, or duodenal atresia in infants. The latter is particularly known for producing the 'two-bubble' appearance in the erect position; distal duodenal obstruction by malrotation of the gut may produce a 'three-bubble' appearance, one each in gastric fundus, antrum and/or duodenal cap and fourth part of the duodenum.

The first two or three loops of the *jejunum* normally lie in the left side of the abdomen above the iliac fossa, and the remainder in the middle; most of the ileum is in the pelvis or just above it. Again, the jejunum and ileum are not visualized unless they contain appreciable quantities of gas, and as a rule only an odd loop can be seen. More gas than usual can be seen in a normal small gut in four conditions, in which it is not significant. It is frequent in crying babies, who swallow vast quantities of air, and in patients who have either been in bed for a few days or have had even a few hours recumbency enforced on them by an acute illness. Acute enteritis also produces an increase of gas in the gut and it may be seen in the abdominal crises of porphyria. But there are three serious conditions in which this is of diagnostic significance. Large amounts of gas are seen in the small gut in acute intestinal obstruction but in order to make a firm diagnosis of this condition it is necessary to show that the gut is *dilated* with gas and air, which means that its diameter must be more than half the width of a lumbar vertebral body. In a supine view, in such a condition only the gas will be seen but in an erect view the gas rises to the top of each distended loop, sometimes forming 'arcades', and horizontal gas-fluid levels can be seen. Similar dilatation also occurs in paralytic ileus which is distinguished from small gut obstruction by the fact that in ileus the colon is usually dilated, also, whereas in obstruction the colon is usually empty or contains normal faecal matter. In subacute or intermittent obstruction the distinction can be very difficult. Another condition which may produce a similar appearance is a mesenteric embolus or thrombus (due to loss of peristalsis from ischaemia), and again differentiation can be difficult, but it is sometimes possible in this condition to show that a segment of the gut wall is thickened and not stretched so thinly as would be expected in an obstructive condition. In very severe acute obstruction the small gut is distended with fluid only, and the abdomen shows only diffuse shadowing of water density − the so-called 'empty abdomen'. In fact, it is over-full, but not with gas! This can also be seen in gangrene of a long loop of small gut. In closed-loop obstruction of the small gut due to volvulus, compression by a band or an internal hernia, the fluid-filled loop resembles a central abdominal mass displacing dilated loops upwards; the so-called 'pseudo-tumour'. In 'gall-stone ileus' the triad of air in the biliary tree, small gut distension and an opacity in the lower abdomen has already been described.

The *colon* is almost always visible throughout

its length because it almost always contains gas, or faecal matter with its typical coarsely speckled appearance, or both (*Figure 3.5*). It can in most cases be seen through dilated loops of small gut and should be looked for carefully. In general, it lies more peripherally than small gut which tends to be more central.

The *caecum,* while usually in the right iliac fossa, may be anywhere from the pelvis to the liver, but the hepatic flexure can practically

gas may be seen. Frequently, the *sigmoid colon,* which normally lies within the pelvis, is enlarged in all these conditions of general enlargement and displacement upwards of the other parts of the colon results; this is also seen in megacolon, in patients with an unusually long sigmoid and in sigmoid volvulus. Distension of the caecum with a fluid level may be seen in caecal volvulus, producing a large gas shadow with a fluid level. It often lies in the RIF but may appear to arise

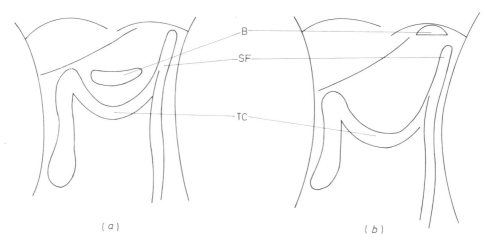

Figure 3.5   Diagrams showing the differing relationships of the gastric air-bubble (B) to the transverse colon (TC) and the splenic flexure (SF) of the colon in (a) supine and (b) erect views of the abdomen.

always be identified below the edge of the liver and the right costal margin. The transverse colon loops down, across, and then up to the splenic flexure which is higher than the hepatic flexure, frequently being up against the left diaphragm. The *descending colon* is almost always visible although it may be represented only by a thin, perhaps discontinuous, channel of gas.

It follows that displacements of the colon by masses are easily visualized, and obstructive lesions may often be localized by noticing normal but collapsed colon distal to, and dilated colon proximal to, the lesion. The grossly dilated toxic colon of an acute ulcerative colitis is readily recognizable, since the whole colon is involved in gaseous distension with thin walls; in the dilatation due to Hirschsprung's disease in children, the dilated colon is full of faecal matter; in older patients with chronic constipation the colon frequently contains much faecal matter, and in the atonic dilatation of old age considerable distension with

from the pelvis. The presence of distended small gut but a collapsed remainder of colon distinguishes it from the sigmoid volvulus arising out of the pelvis.

An important lesion to identify in a plain film is that due to localized ischaemic disease of the colon, usually in the upper part of the descending colon — a 3–5 cm segment — narrowed in a somewhat scalloped fashion (so-called 'thumb-printing') due to localized mucosal oedema. A large inferior mesenteric infarct, on the other hand, eventually produces generalized widespread small and large gut dilatation.

In the severe infective condition of necrotizing enterocolitis of infancy the colon contains gas but because the mucosa separates from the wall a fine double shadow can be seen, particularly in a supine view of the descending colon.

Abnormalities of hollow organs and the pancreas are to be found in *Plates 3.17–3.32*; systematic scrutiny, particularly of gas shadows, is essential.

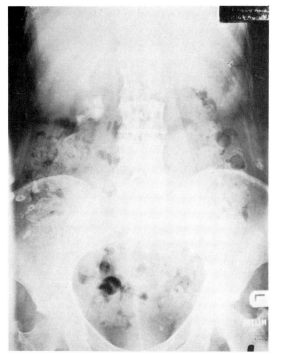

Plate 3.17

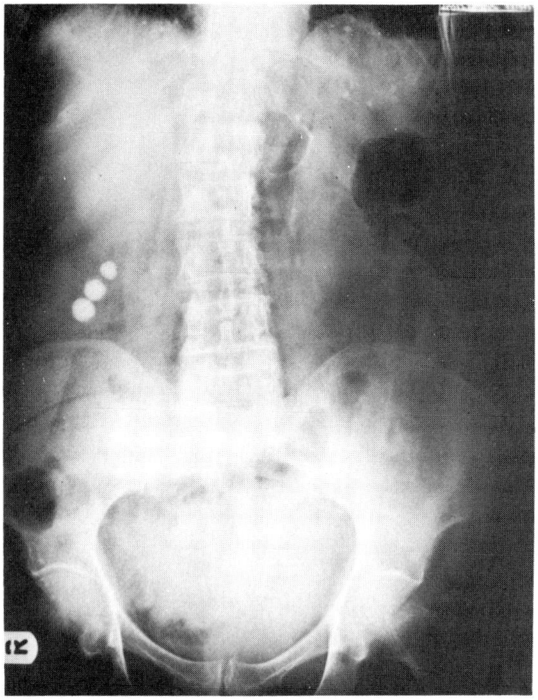

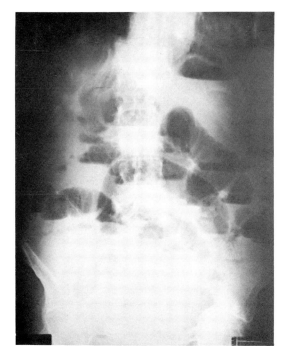

Plate 3.19

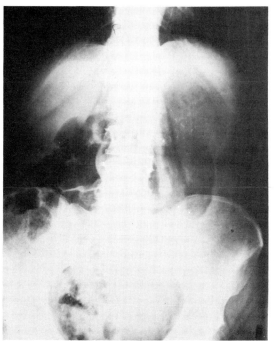

Plate 3.18

Plate 3.20

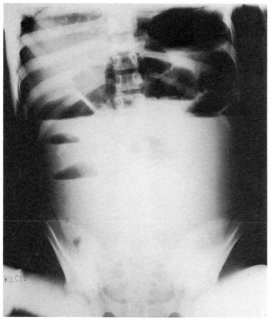

Plate 3.21

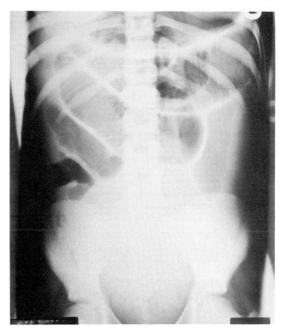

Plate 3.22

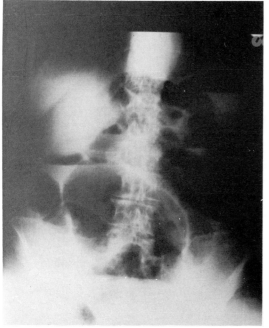

Plate 3.23

Plate 3.24

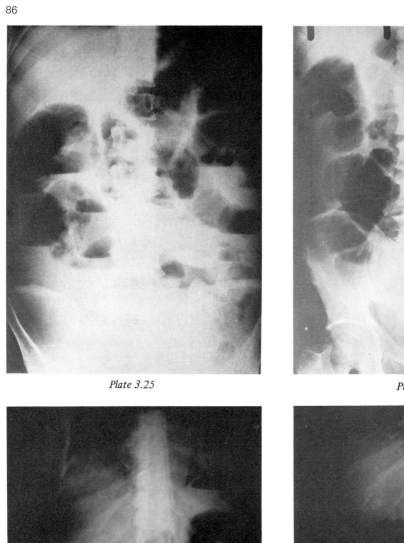

Plate 3.25

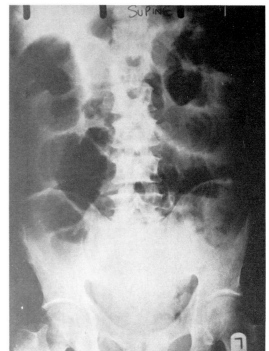

Plate 3.26

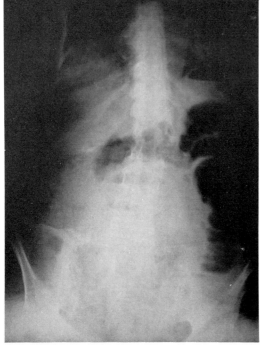
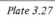

Plate 3.27

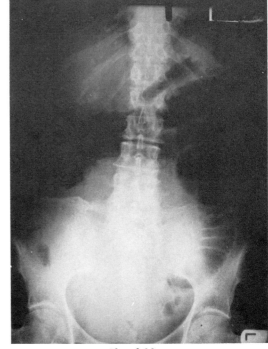

Plate 3.28

87

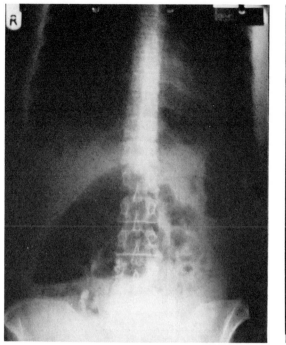

Plate 3.29

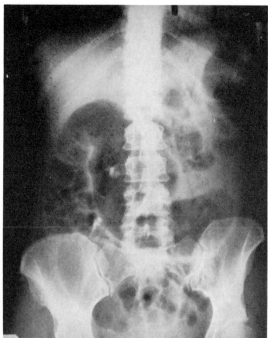

Plate 3.30

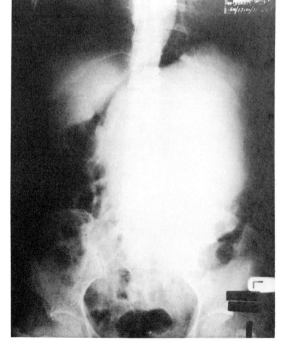

Plate 3.31

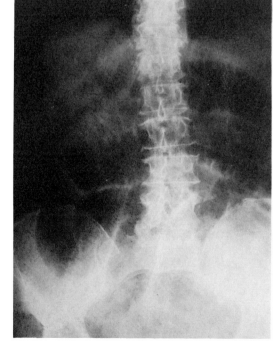

Plate 3.32

SOLUTIONS

Plate 3.17   Staghorn calculus in the right kidney, in two parts. Note also old opaque injections into the buttocks.

Plate 3.18   The row of three opacities to the right of the spine in the position of the gall bladder are gallstones. Note also lumbar scoliosis concave to the left.

Plate 3.19   Dilated loops of the small gut with fluid levels seen in the erect position, the gastric air-bubble being seen separately beneath the left diaphragm. The colon is not obvious here. This looks like an acute obstruction. To find the cause it is necessary to look beneath the right inguinal ligament, where a small gas shadow indicates an obstructed hernia, probably femoral.

Plate 3.20   Fine dots extending for a short distance to the right of the spine and rather more over to the left are due to calcification in the pancreas.

Plate 3.21   Erect view of the abdomen of a child showing dilated loops of gut with gas–fluid levels. In the right iliac fossa can be seen a somewhat flattened group of gas shadows which, being in the position of the caecum, are most likely to represent that organ containing normal gas and faecal matter.

Plate 3.22   Supine view of the same abdomen as in Plate 3.21. Dilated loops of gut in the upper abdomen, with the dilated stomach full of gas above them. The same collection of flattened shadows can be seen in the right iliac fossa, medial to the extraperitoneal fat line, and again look like caecum. This must therefore be an obstructive lesion of the small gut proximal to the caecum. At operation it proved to be a band across the base of a loop.

Plate 3.23   Erect view of the abdomen showing dilated loops of gut and a particularly large loop apparently arising out of the pelvis with a gas–fluid level. No obvious colon shadows.

Plate 3.24   Supine view of the same abdomen as in Plate 3.23; although the gas-filled loop arising from the pelvis is not completely shown, it is still in the same position. All the gas-filled dilated loops of gut in the remainder of the abdomen appear to be about the same size and there is no obvious distended colon shadow which would have been expected if this were a volvulous of the sigmoid. In fact, it was a volvulus of the caecum; the variability in position of the caecum must not be forgotten, and it frequently lies in the pelvis.

Plate 3.25   Erect view of the abdomen, showing dilated loops of gut with gas–fluid levels. The loops are not obviously identifiable as either large or small gut, particularly on the right, but it is possible to see some irregular shadowing which looks like faecal matter.

Plate 3.26   Supine view of the same abdomen as in Plate 3.25; most of the dilated loops of gut now look more like small gut and there appears to be normal faecal matter in the transverse and descending colon. This thus suggests either an obstruction distal to the hepatic flexure of the colon, if the dilated gut on the right is colon, or in the ileum if it is in fact small gut. At operation it proved to be the latter.

Plate 3.27   Erect view of the abdomen showing dilated gut on the left, a normal gastric air-bubble, and an apparent mass in the middle of the abdomen, but including some shallow gas–fluid levels in its upper part. On the right can be seen what appears to be normal caecum and ascending colon, and the transverse colon is displaced upwards, but there is also some dilated gut here.

Plate 3.28   Supine view of the same abdomen as in Plate 3.27. The central 'mass' is again well shown, with dilated gut displaced upwards and outwards. The appearances on both films together are highly suggestive of a closed loop small gut obstruction, producing the so-called 'pseudo-tumour' appearance, with dilated small gut proximal to the obstructed loop and normal (invisible) small gut distal to it, with a normal caecum.

SOLUTIONS

Plate 3.29 Erect view of the abdomen showing a large dilated loop of gut on the right with a gas–fluid level and another, less extensive, loop in the left upper quadrant. There are some less dilated loops of gut elsewhere. A small gastric air-bubble can be seen beneath the left diaphragm.

Plate 3.30 Supine view of the same abdomen as on Plate 3.29. It is now fairly clear that the greatly dilated loops are large intestine and the others the small gut; but the descending colon is barely visible. This was acute-on-chronic obstruction of the colon, due to carcinoma involving the descending colon at the splenic flexure. Note that the small gut is less distended than in the cases where the site of obstruction was in the small gut itself.

Plate 3.31 Large mass in the middle of the abdomen, a little to the left, elevating the stomach, displacing stomach and duodenum to the right and depressing the colon downwards. This was a pancreatic cyst. The alternatives are some other retroperitoneal tumour, renal tumour, cyst or dilated collecting system, or just possibly aneurysm, but this pattern of separation of stomach and colon is classically seen in pancreatic cyst.

Plate 3.32 Supine view of the abdomen, showing several greatly dilated loops of small gut. The colon is not visible so that this is most likely to be a small gut obstruction. There is no obvious thickening of the walls therefore acute ischaemic disease is less likely. The diagnosis is made by looking at the solid organs and then at the hollow organs in order, when it becomes clear that the dark shadows in the liver area are due to gas in a dilated biliary tree. This is gallstone ileus.

Pelvic organs

SIGMOID COLON

The sigmoid colon may be invisible or may contain faecal matter and/or gas, when it is usually traceable as a continuation of the descending colon. It is not normally possible to visualize the different folds or loops (for which barium enema will be needed), but if it contains much faecal matter the whole pelvis seems to show the characteristic speckled appearance. Diverticula are occasionally seen as rows of small, rounded, gas shadows 3–5 mm in diameter, or as opacities if there has been a barium meal or enema within the last week or two; the barium residues in them may be very persistent. If the diverticula have been infected or there is a peri-diverticular abscess there may be some increase in general density of the pelvic contents, but it is a non-specific appearance having other causes (other pelvic abscesses, cysts or neoplastic masses). If the sigmoid is longer than usual, it may be possible to see its loop arising out of the pelvis; and if it twists on itself to produce a sigmoid volvulus the greatly dilated loop with a fluid level in each limb has a characteristic appearance — it may almost fill the whole abdomen. It is distinguished from caecal volvulus by the presence of dilated descending, transverse and ascending colon proximal to it.

RECTUM

Again, the rectum contains either gas or faecal matter but its outline is often easier to make out than the sigmoid, being midline and lower down. Sometimes crescents of gas can be seen on one or both sides of the faecal matter. The rectum may be displaced by other masses in the pelvis.

Infants swallow and pass a lot of air. The rectum is therefore normally full of gas, which can be best demonstrated by taking a lateral view with the baby held upside down by its legs. In imperforate anus it is important to know the depth from the skin surface at which the anal canal is closed, and the 'upside-down lateral' view, with an opaque marker on the anal dimple, is of great value.

BLADDER

The soft-tissue shadow of the bladder is often distinguishable from the other pelvic contents, because it is of water density and there are traces of fat in the fascia surrounding it, particularly in the female. Empty, it shows only as a flat oval shadow just behind the pubis in the male and just above it in the female (on account of the differing pelvic inclination) when it also commonly shows a shallow depression in its roof, produced by the normal uterus. When full it shows as a dense rounded shadow and when greatly distended it may reach into the abdomen, even above the level of the umbilicus, which is about the level of L4–5. It is sometimes difficult, at first glance in the female, to know whether such a shadow is an ovarian cyst or a large bladder. In the former case, careful scrutiny will often disclose a narrow transradiant band separating the bladder from the cyst above it; the bladder will, of course, have a different shape after being emptied if films are taken before and after micturition or catheterization.

Opaque stones of varying sizes occur in the bladder, either round and single, or multiple and faceted. The latter change position between supine and erect views, a useful diagnostic feature, and a single one may also show some movement if not too large. Foreign bodies in the bladder become calcified with recognizable or bizarre shapes. In the male, calculi may form in an enlarged prostate gland, showing as a collection of small (1–2 mm) dense opacities behind or just above the pubis. The bladder may also calcify in bilharzia infection (schistosomiasis), producing fine dense curvilinear streaks in the bladder walls; malignancy occurs in a small but appreciable portion of these cases. Calcification can occur in malignant papillomata. All these opacities have to be distinguished from calcified lymph glands or iliac vessels, pelvic phleboliths and stones in the lower ureters (or even, rarely, a stone in the renal pelvis of an ectopic kidney), and intravenous urography usually solves the problem if it is not possible on a plain film.

MALE AND FEMALE ORGANS

Male   The shadows of the external genitalia are occasionally confusing if not identified. The seminal vesicles are sometimes calcified and rise remarkably high in the pelvis, above the level of the ischial spines, due either to tuberculous or bilharzia infection or, rarely, associated with long-standing diabetes.

Female   The vagina is normally invisible but a freshly inserted vaginal tampon, consisting of loose absorbent cotton wool and therefore largely of air density, shows as a transradiant oblong, lying slightly obliquely in the lower part of the pelvis. As it absorbs blood, it will assume water density and lose its outline. Ring pessaries of various types may be seen. The uterus, being of water density, is not seen normally but all intra-uterine contraceptive devices are radio-opaque and are easily recognized. They are sometimes extra-uterine. A bulky uterus may produce a soft-tissue shadow above the bladder and a pregnant uterus will be recognizable at 10—14 weeks. All that may be seen of the fetus in early pregnancy is a single curvilinear shadow of part of the skull vault, the rest of the small bony shadows being concealed over the bones of the maternal pelvis; and to identify this will need very careful scrutiny.

What will be very obvious is calcification in a uterine fibroid and these as a rule vary from 1—5 cm in diameter. The appearance is of a roughly rounded, slightly irregular and craggy dense shadow, often midline but possibly asymmetrical above the bladder shadow, more regular than a calcified tuberculous gland but more irregular than a bladder stone. Occasionally there is more than one, of different sizes. The distinction can sometimes be difficult on a plain film; a lateral view may help.

The Fallopian tubes and ovaries are not visible when normal but ovarian cysts or tumours produce shadows of water density, asymmetrical originally. A cyst may, however, grow to a great size and may even reach up to fill the whole abdomen and mimic ascites, but gas-filled loops of gut will be distributed centrifugally round the cyst with little change in position between erect and supine views, allowing differentiation from ascites (*see* page 66). A dermoid cyst of the ovary may be recognized by the presence of a tooth or two within the soft-tissue shadow, which may not be obvious. Such a cyst contains much sebeceous material which is nearer to the density of fat so that radiographically it may be of less than water density. A tubal abscess or hydrosalpinx may show an asymmetrical pelvic shadow and some such appearance may be seen in a ruptured ectopic pregnancy (though it would be a bold man to diagnose the latter condition radiologically).

Some typical pelvic lesions are shown in *Plates 3.33—3.41.*

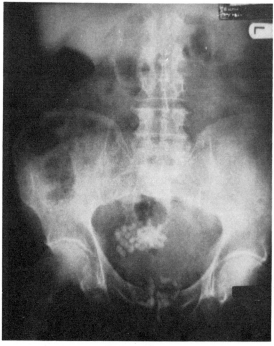

Plate 3.33

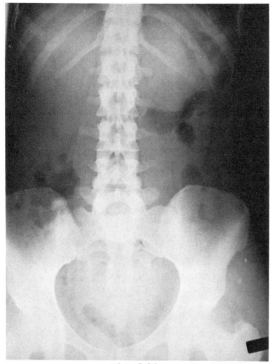
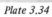

Plate 3.34

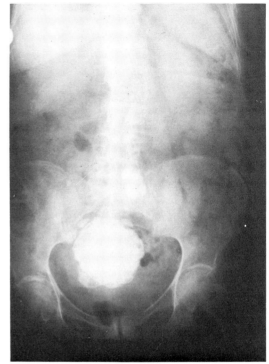

Plate 3.35

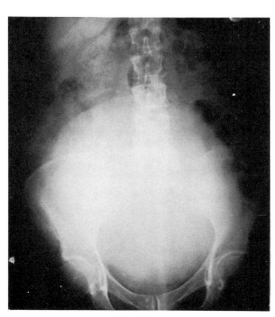

Plate 3.36

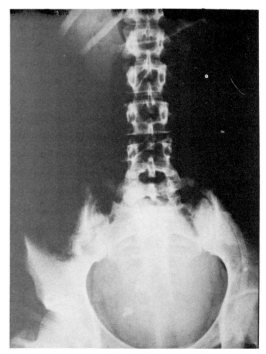

Plate 3.37

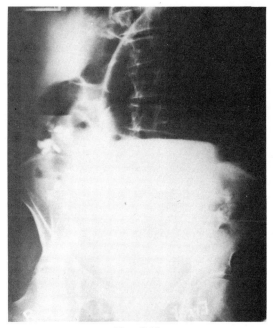

Plate 3.38

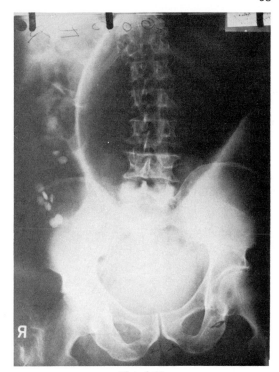

Plate 3.39

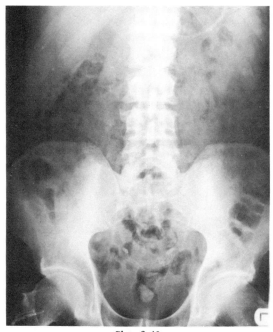

Plate 3.40

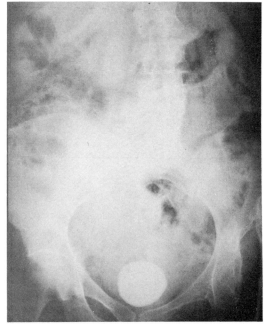

Plate 3.41

SOLUTIONS

Plate 3.33 *There is a collection of small dense opacities in the upper part of the pelvis to the right, and another collection lower down, partly behind the pubis and rather more irregular. The lower group is typical in site and appearance of prostatic calculi, and the upper group are stones in the bladder, elevated by the enlarged prostate, only the lower part of which contains calcareous matter. Plate 3.42 confirms this, showing the bladder contents opacified by intravenous urography.*

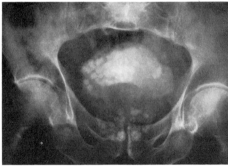

Plate 3.42

Plate 3.34 *An oblong shadow of air density lies obliquely in the lower part of the pelvis — typical appearance of a vaginal tampon.*

Plate 3.35 *An irregular, dense, roughly rounded mass lies in the lower part of the pelvis. It is not as smooth or as regular as the bladder stone seen in Plate 3.41 and is a uterine fibroid. Note also a lumbar scoliosis concave to right with osteoarthritic changes, and another dense shadow above the fibroid. This may be either another fibroid or a calcified gland.*

Plate 3.36 *There is some relatively ill-defined dense shadowing arising out of the pelvis, displacing the normal sigmoid gas shadows. It is just possible to make out a roughly linear transradiant shadow across the lower third of the pelvis; this is due to fat in the fascia separating the bladder below from the mass above. In a female, this is most likely to be an ovarian cyst or tumour.*

Plate 3.37 *There is a rounded mass in the pelvis, and it is just possible to make out the flattened bladder beneath it. Two dense opacities can be seen within the mass, their shape being consistent with teeth. This is the typical appearance of a dermoid cyst. A longer, curvilinear shadow above and to the left of the pelvis appears to be a catheter, perhaps passed to empty the bladder and so distinguish it from the cyst.*

Plate 3.38 *Erect view of the abdomen showing a greatly enlarged hollow viscus with a gas−fluid level arising out of the pelvis, with other dilated gut gas shadows above and to the right, also showing gas−fluid levels. A collection of dense opacities looks like tablets in the gut which from its position should be caecum.*

Plate 3.39 *Supine view of the same abdomen as in Plate 3.38. The enlarged gas-filled gut shadow is again seen, and there is nothing to suggest normal colon anywhere. The tablets in what should be dilated caecum are again seen. This is the typical appearance of a volvulus of the sigmoid colon, with obstruction of the colon proximal to it.*

Plate 3.40 *A pair of calcified, apparently tubular structures, rather like a pair of antlers, can be seen in the middle on the pelvis. This is the typical appearance of calcified seminal vesicles, in this case in a man with long-standing diabetes.*

Plate 3.41 *Dense rounded shadow with smooth edges in the pelvis. Lumbar scoliosis concave to right and some disorganization of the hip joint. This was a bladder stone.*

Abnormal and unanatomical shadows (the 'rag-bag')

Once the basic structures and the organs have been visualized — or found wanting — on the radiograph, it is then essential to look over the film again and see if there are any other shadows not accounted for. These may be diagnostic, or at least offer a clue to the diagnosis and are, of course, much easier to see and perceive if all the other shadows have been identified. Such extra shadows may be classified by their radiographic density — air, fat, water or bone — and some information gained by considering their location. Again, it must be doubly checked that they are not due to a normal or distorted normal shadow in an unusual location.

GAS-SHADOWS

Intraperitoneal In certain locations small collections of gas can be diagnostic. Free gas beneath the diaphragms has already been considered. A short crescentic shadow not more than 2 cm in length against the lower liver margin, is likely to be due to a perforated duodenal ulcer. A gas shadow with a fluid level medial to the gastric air-bubble, but just behind it in a lateral view, is likely to be in an abscess in the lesser sac. Gas may also collect in the pouch of Rutherford Morrison, beneath the liver.

Retroperitoneal Small collections of rounded gas-bubbles up to 5 mm size, in areas of the abdomen where gas-bubbles would not be expected (for example, medial to the descending colon, over the psoas shadows or in the upper left quadrant) may be due to retroperitoneal abscess cavities. Their distinguishing feature from gut shadows is their failure to change position between erect and supine views.

Peri-visceral Gas-shadows may be seen in relation to any of the hollow organs and usually denote some sort of inflammatory condition with a gas-forming organism, for example, emphysema gangrenosa of the gall bladder, or a similar infection of the stomach, but the commonest lesion of this type is a pericolic abscess due either to a ruptured diverticulum or to a leak from the region of a carcinoma. Such an abscess may even point on the surface of the abdomen. Diverticula themselves can contain air, but a well-marked row of gas-shadows close to and indenting the colon is due to gas cysts in the wall — the rather rare condition known as pneumatosis cystoides intestinalis, or intestinal pneumatosis. Many small gas-shadows

with fluid levels in the erect position may be seen in diverticulosis of the small gut.

Boundaries Gas-shadows in the abdominal walls may be in abscess cavities, and the very rare spigelian hernia between the layers may produce them. Surgical emphysema may be seen, perhaps tracking down from the chest. Inguinal and femoral herniae may contain gas-shadows beneath the inguinal ligament, even right down into the scrotum.

FAT-SHADOWS

Shadows more transradiant than the solid organs may be cast by collections of fatty material such as lipoma (for example, retroperitoneal or sub-cutaneous), liposarcoma (for example, of kidney) or dermoid cysts, but the subcutaneous lipoma may be confusing since it is often partly calcified.

SHADOWS OF WATER DENSITY

A dense solid-looking mass in the abdomen should be first carefully checked for continuity with solid organs — thus, it may be a liver or renal tumour or an odd-shaped enlarged spleen — and for origin from the pelvis, particularly in the female. Its relationship to the hollow organs should also be considered since it might be one of these full of fluid, as in a greatly distended renal pelvis or a closed loop obstruction of small gut. If it is none of these, its location can sometimes be inferred from displacement of other organs; in particular, anything displacing either the kidney or the duodenum is likely to be a retroperitoneal tumour or other space-occupying lesion; for example, a large tumour or cyst of the pancreas classically displaces the stomach upwards, widens the duodenal loop and displaces the colon downwards. Aortic aneurysms commonly have calcified rims but not always, and again may mimic a retroperitoneal tumour. Lateral displacement of a psoas outline generally indicates a psoas abscess, often tuberculous, even in the absence of vertebral lesions.

CALCIFICATIONS AND OTHER HIGH-DENSITY SHADOWS

Unidentified calcifications can be most confusing. If they do not fit into the normally expected location of the various organs, the possibility of enlargement or displacement should be considered; for example, calcification in a renal tumour in an enlarged kidney or, indeed, in a kidney misshapen by tuberculous infection, or perhaps an adrenal tumour. All tumours may occasionally calcify (particularly in children) and retroperitoneal tumours, tumours of the biliary tract or tumours of bone or fibrous tissue may be suspected. Calcification close to the lumbar spine, particularly if associated with a disturbed psoas outline, is strongly suggestive of tuberculous disease of the vertebrae. Calcified parasites may be seen, such as the oval 2 x 4 mm shadows of cysticercosis, long axes in the lines of muscle fibres between which they lie, or the coils of dots, sometimes coalescent, due to guinea-worms (*Dracunculus medinensis*) in the fascial planes between muscles. Small C-shaped calcifications on the peritoneal surfaces of any organ, and scattered through the peritoneum are likely to be due to the tongue-worm (*Armiller armillatus*) found in Central and West Africa and some other tropical areas.

Other high-density shadows may be due to foreign bodies. In the gut they can usually be recognized by some well-known shape such as coins, pins, spoons, thermometer fragments, toy soldiers, etc., and by their relationship to the gut shadows, since they will usually have been swallowed, accidentally or as a result of mental aberration. The eating of soil or other forms of pica may lead to large quantities of small opacities appearing in the colon, and lead shot may be seen in those in the habit of eating game birds. Foreign bodies not in the gut may be missiles or metallic fragments from explosions or machinery, traffic or other accidents, or sharp objects such as needles which have pierced the skin or gut and migrated; they may appear in any part of the abdomen. Windscreen glass is also often opaque and produces typical small quadrilateral shadows.

An important type of high density shadow to identify is that due to old injections into the buttocks, since it may give a useful clue to previous disease; for example, bismuth for syphilis, quinine for malaria. Bismuth is seen in longitudinal streaks in the line of the gluteal muscle fibres, and quinine produces oval rounded opacities about 1−2 cm in diameter. Other substances produce less specific appearances.

Plates 3.43−3.47 which follow this section are not intended to be easy, but if the material in the previous sections has been of any value to the reader, systemic scrutiny should enable a reasonable deduction to be made about the probable location of the lesion and some reasonable alternative aetiological solutions offered.

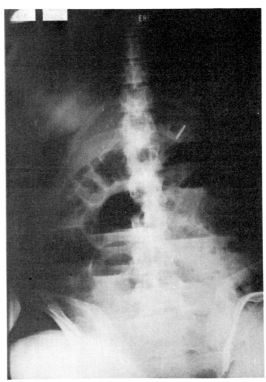

Plate 3.43   Post-operative abdominal pain and swelling

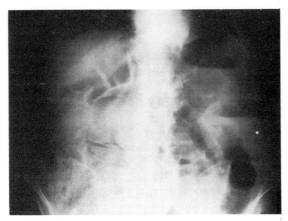

Plate 3.44   Pain and swelling left side of abdomen

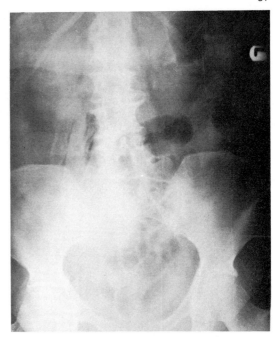

Plate 3.45   Abdominal pain, more marked on right

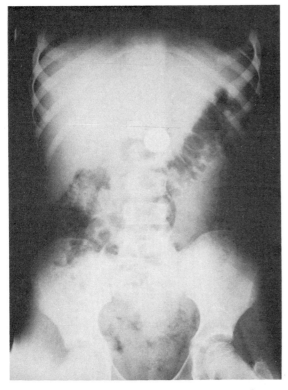

Plate 3.46   Patient lost a marble. Where is it?

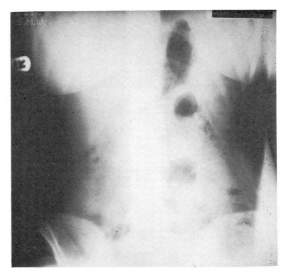

Plate 3.47   Road traffic accident. Left-sided pain, slight shock

SOLUTIONS

Plate 3.43   Post-operative erect film following re-implantation of the left ureter into the bladder. Dilated loops of small gut with gas–fluid levels and also some dilatation of the colon. This is likely to be a paralytic ileus. In addition there is a collection of small gas shadows to the left of the lower lumbar spine, of the type seen in retro-peritoneal abscesses. In fact, there had been a small leak of urine into this region alongside the ureter during the operation. Note opaque tip of gastric tube in left hypochondrium.

Plate 3.44   Erect view of the abdomen showing unusual gas-shadows. That beneath the left dia-phragm is likely to be the gastric air-bubble with its gas–fluid level; a kinked gas-shadow lying across the upper abdomen is likely to be the transverse colon; another unusual gas-shadow with a gas–fluid level in the left side of the abdomen is difficult to identify, but below it a roughly vertical gas-shadow is in the position of the descending colon, narrowing irregularly at its upper end. This suggests that the pathology lies in the splenic flexure of the colon; the unusual gas-shadow was due to a peri-colic abscess pointing on the surface of the abdomen, associated with a carcinoma of the splenic flexure.

Plate 3.45   Linear gas-shadows can be seen in the line of the right psoas muscle. Other gut gas-shadows look slightly more dilated than usual but not enough to suggest acute obstruction. Some increased shadowing of water density over the right side of the sacrum. Lumbar scoliosis concave to left with O.A. changes. The gas-shadows along the psoas suggest serious retroperitoneal involvement, prob-ably in the right iliac fossa or overlying the right sacral ala — either an abscess with gas-forming organisms or some lesion allowing gas to escape retroperitoneally from the gut. This was found at operation to be due to a carcinoma of the caecum with invasion of the ilio-psoas muscle.

Plate 3.46   Dense round shadow in the middle of the upper abdomen, overlying the shadow of the gastric air-bubble in the pyloric antrum (supine film). This young patient had swallowed a marble and it now appears to be in the pyloric antrum of the stomach.

Plate 3.47   Supine view of the abdomen. Neither diaphragms nor pelvis are shown. The gas-shadows of the splenic flexure and the descending colon are displaced medially by a large haematoma in the upper left paravertebral gutter due to a ruptured spleen. Note breast shadows overlying the upper abdomen; the tip of the spleen has also been displaced downwards.

CHAPTER 4

The Bones

Bone radiology is much more complex than is generally supposed. In order to convey a relatively simple scheme for looking at a bone radiograph, it has proved necessary to include much detail to explain the necessity for the scheme and for reference.

There is rarely any value in studying a single bone in isolation from surrounding soft tissue, or from other bones. Bone disease may be localized or generalized. With localized bone lesions the surrounding soft tissue may be involved, for example, soft-tissue damage in fractures, oedema completely surrounding acute osteomyelitis and the soft-tissue masses often associated with malignant disease of bone. Generalized bone disease may involve all bones, some bones only, even a single bone, either in intrinsic bone disease or where the bone lesion is merely one facet of a general disease. Examples are osteomalacia with pseudo-fractures in predictable sites such as the ribs, the axillary border of the scapula, the pubic rami or the medial cortex of the femur; the multiple fractures of different ages in the 'battered baby' syndrome or in osteogenesis imperfecta; the scattered asymmetrical lesions of Paget's disease or fibrous dysplasia; the occasional single bone cyst of hyperparathyroidism; the generalized bone changes of haemoglobinopathies; and the multiple or single metastases of malignant disease. In addition, therefore, to systematic study of the whole film, thought must also be given to the possible necessity to radiograph other parts of the body. There are standard skeletal surveys which will include the bones most commonly involved in generalized disease on a reasonable number of films.

RADIOGRAPHY

It is essential to check the radiography of bone as elsewhere, particularly the marking and the side. Position should be assessed from anatomical knowledge of the bone, and the quality should be such as to show both soft-tissue outlines and trabecular pattern. There are conventional radiographic positions, outside the scope of this book for detailed discussion, with which the student will become familiar.

Scheme of scrutiny

The scheme to be adopted for the scrutiny of bones is again anatomical, but so simplified that it is essential that the detailed normal anatomy be checked at each stage. If each bone is regarded as an irregular quadrilateral with excrescences, then in long bones the shafts account for two sides and the bone ends, forming the joints, for the other two. In other bones, analogous concepts can be applied. This allows for a simple scheme which falls into threes — the soft tissues, the bones and the joints. Each of these subdivides into three, and some subdivide still further, as shown in *Table 4.1*.

In many cases a final diagnosis will not be possible, but it is usually helpful to try to place a lesion in one of the following aetiological groups (the so-called 'surgical sieve').

Congenital	Neoplastic
Traumatic	Degenerative
Inflammatory	Metabolic
Vascular	Miscellaneous

Table 4.1

SCRUTINY OF BONE RADIOGRAPHS

I Soft tissues	II Bones	III Joints

(1) Transradiancies
(2) Masses
(3) Calcifications
	(1) Periosteum
	  (a) Type of reaction
	  (b) Distribution
	  (c) Associated lesions
	(2) Cortex
	  (a) Continuity
	  (b) Thickness
	  (c) Density
	(3) Medulla
	  (a) Trabeculae
	  (b) Defects
	  (c) Calcification
		(1) Soft tissues
		  (a) Peri-articular tissue
		  (b) Capsule and ligaments
		  (c) Joint space
		(2) Bone ends
		  (a) Subarticular cortex
		  (b) Joint margins
		  (c) Medulla
		(3) Bone ends in childhood
		  (a) Epiphyses
		  (b) Epiphyseal line
		  (c) Metaphysis

SOFT TISSUES

A strong light may be needed to see the anatomy of the soft tissues since they are often dark on films taken to show bone detail. Skin edges, superficial fascia (transradiant due to its fat content) and muscle layers separated by deep fascia should be seen, and some tendons are identifiable in lateral views, for example, triceps, patellar and Achilles' tendons. Defects in muscle layers due to wasting or atrophy occur in old neuropathies, including poliomyelitis, nerve injuries and some congenital conditions.

Transradiancies

Dark shadows representing gas, distinguishable from fascial layers of fat may be seen in surgical emphysema, in gas gangrene and where injury has allowed air to enter tissue planes or joint spaces. A larger transradiancy of fat density displacing other tissues can be produced by a lipoma, although these sometimes contain fibrous strands and calcification due to fat necrosis.

Masses

A well-defined shadow of similar density to that of muscle may be due to a benign tumour or a localized inflammatory lesion. Varicose veins should be recognized if large enough, and sometimes contain phleboliths. Malignant tumours usually have less well-defined edges and may only be recognized by the displacement of a muscle.

Inflammatory disease tends to be associated with oedema which conceals the fascial planes, so that all soft-tissue architecture may be lost in the area of a localized cellulitis. In early acute osteomyelitis, soft-tissue oedema is seen all around the bone which may look otherwise normal, since bone changes may not occur for 10—14 days.

Calcifications

Soft-tissue calcifications may be incidental and irrelevant, but are sometimes diagnostic. Most occur in damaged or necrotic tissue but metabolic factors may also operate.

Traumatic calcified lesions include haematomata and scar tissue, the dense streaks in muscles known as myositis ossificans being due to tears which first calcify and then ossify, the thin lines of calcification being due to partial tendinous or ligamentous tears (for example, the Pellegrini—Steida lesion parallel to the medial femoral condyle) and the fine calcifications alongside the finger tendons, probably due to chronic irritation, known as peritendinitis calcarea.

Tuberculosis is the most likely cause of calcification near to an infected joint or vertebral body, the para-spinal cold abscess. Some tropical parasites calcify on death in the tissues and can be recognized. Cysticerci, *Armillifer armillatus* and guinea-worms have been mentioned in Chapter 3; the latter can occasionally act as nidus for a sterile abscess forming a soft-tissue mass of water density with calcification near one edge. Filariae may be seen as long threads, especially in the fingers.

Phleboliths are common in vascular lesions, varicose veins and angiomatous malformations and are often diagnostic.

Calcification in a benign tumour usually suggests chondroma, sometimes hamartoma, but it also occurs in lipoma. Any malignant tumour may calcify, especially in children.

Calcification in bursa or tendon sheath, associated with painful restriction of movement, is best known in the shoulder in supraspinatus tendinitis, but can occur elsewhere (for example, in the triceps). Ectopic calcification is often seen where the blood calcium level is raised, such as in hyperparathyroidism or vitamin D poisoning. In the Ehlers—Danlos syndrome (pseudoxanthoma elasticum) there are fine calcifications beneath the skin. In scleroderma (systemic sclerosis) the fingertips often show calcifications beneath the shrunken skin, often associated with pressure atrophy of the tips of the terminal phalanges.

In paraplegia, with long-standing immobility of the lower limbs, extensive sheets of calcification of muscle round the hip joints may occur, sometimes ossifying; even occasionally round a hemiplegic hip joint.

In parts of Africa collections of dense calcification are seen in the condition known as calcinosis circumscripta (if extensive if may be called calcinosis universalis).

Calcification of blood vessels is common over the age of 65 years, frequently associated with arteriosclerosis and degenerative vascular disease generally, including diabetes, and also in any form of hypercalcaemia.

Other causes of local tissue necrosis followed by calcification, or of ectopic calcification, may well come to light, so that the foregoing is not an exhaustive list.

Some soft-tissue lesions will be found in *Plates 4.1—4.5.*

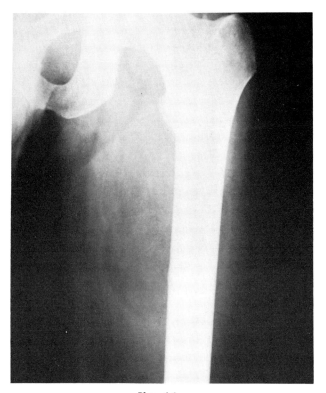

Plate 4.1

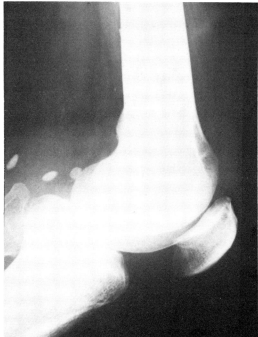

Plate 4.2

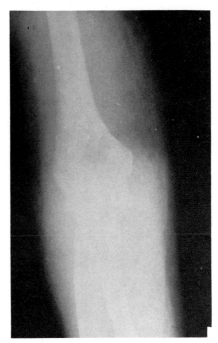

Plate 4.3

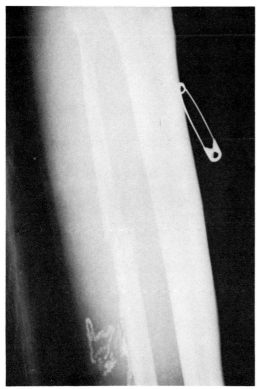

Plate 4.4

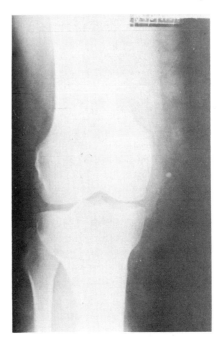

Plate 4.5

SOLUTIONS

Plate 4.1   In the middle of the thigh and overlying the femur, there is a large, lobulated and relatively transradiant mass, displacing the muscle bundles medially. Any soft-tissue mass can do this but the relative transradiancy suggests fat. This was a large lipoma.

Plate 4.2   Behind the knee joint and overlying the femur are small oval dense opacities, their long axes lying in the line of the muscles. These are typical of cysticercosis, and represent the dead parasites.

Plate 4.3   Loss of the normal skin, fascial and muscular outlines in the medial part of the upper arm, above the elbow, although the anatomy is normal elsewhere; there is instead an irregular coarse network with obvious swelling. This is typical of oedema and in this case was due to a localized cellulitis.

Plate 4.4   Right tibia and fibula with a fracture of the latter in a West African. An incidental finding is a calcified guinea-worm in the lower part of the calf. (The safety pin was in the bandage securing the splint.)

Plate 4.5   On the medial aspect of the lower thigh, knee joint and lower leg, there is, between the skin and the muscle bundles, an irregular, somewhat lobulated soft-tissue structure, with a dense spot by the femoral condyle. This is due to varicose veins and the dense spot is a phlebolith.

BONES

Commence the scrutiny with a general look at the anatomy: a manual of anatomy, a set of normal bone films and a set of dry bones will be useful. First, determine the age group. Childrens' bones have epiphyses and metaphyses and the various excrescences take time to develop. Young adult and middle-aged peoples' bones are well-formed, especially mens, women's bones tending to be more slender, and old peoples' bones are generally thin, particularly those of old women who tend to become progressively more osteoporotic.

Secondly, assess the general size and shape, particularly in relation to the rest of the body and the age. A bone may be too small because of a congenital deformity (for example, that caused by thalidomide, or other embryopathy), or failure to grow due to trauma, neuropathy, disuse atrophy or epiphyseal damage. Enlargement is rare but occurs in some cases of chronic hyperaemia, as in a slow-healing fracture, chronic infection, angiomatous malformation and haemophilia (near deformed joints due to recurrent haemarthroses). It may also occur following infantile cortical hyperostosis and in neurofibromatosis of bone, fibrous dysplasia and Paget's disease.

Variations in shape in the absence of local acquired disease usually indicate congenital bone disease. The commonest cause of symmetrical short thick bones is achondroplasia, proximal limb bones being most affected. Some other rarer bone dystrophies produce more distal shortening, as in the chondro-ectodermal dysplasia of Ellis and van Crefeld, with its delayed appearance of the upper tibial epiphysis.

Thirdly, check the normal anatomical features of the bone to determine that nothing is missing and that there is nothing extra. It often helps to rotate a dry bone in front of the viewing box to check the outline. At this point one should notice anomalies such as a vertebral pedicle or spinous process destroyed by neoplasm, an avulsion fracture of malleolus or tuberosity, or loss of a carpal bone, a digit or a phalanx. Additional structures such as ecchondromata, exostoses, osteomata (single, or multiple as in diaphyseal aclasia), osteophytes of osteo-arthritis, spurs due to old fractures or even additional digits (for example, a sixth digit is seen in chondro-ectodermal dysplasia).

Plates 4.6–4.9 offer some elementary problems in anatomical observation.

The bone should then be examined from without inwards, looking at the periosteum, the cortex and the medulla.

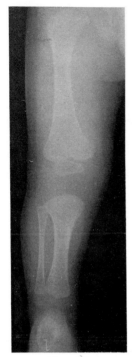

Plate 4.6

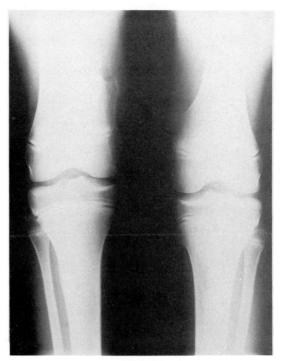

Plate 4.7

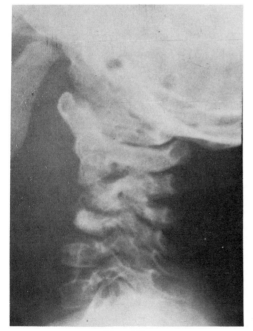

Plate 4.8

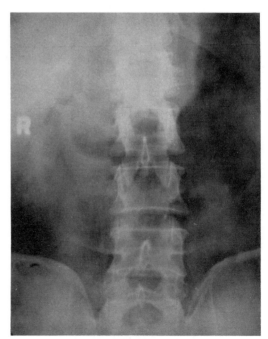

Plate 4.9

SOLUTIONS

Plate 4.6   Right leg of a toddler. Note that the tibia and fibula are relatively short and that the upper tibial epiphysis, normally present at birth, is absent. Clearly, some disturbance of growth and development is present, and this should lead to a search for a congenital bone disease possessing the features seen. It is the chondro-ectodermal dysplasia of Ellis and van Crefeld, which also has impaired general growth and nail and tooth dysplasia.

Plate 4.7   AP view of both knees, showing exostoses arising from the medial aspects of both femoral condyles, and pointing upwards. There is also a flatter exostosis arising from the medial part of the left tibia, tending to point downwards. All these arise from the diaphysis or shaft near to the metaphysis; note that this is a young person in whom growth is not yet complete. These appearances are characteristic of the condition of multiple exostoses or diaphyseal aclasia; eventually all the metaphyseal regions of the long bones will show this type of abnormality.

Plate 4.8   Lateral view of the cervical spine of a child. If care is taken to identify the axis and atlas vertebra and then to count the spinous processes and vertebral bodies downwards, it will be seen that there are seven spinous processes but only apparently six vertebral bodies, (counting atlas and axis as two). The bodies of C3 and C4 are fused and the disc space between C4 and C5 is narrowed; the bodies of C3, C4 and C5 also appear slightly flattened and denser. This is due to tuberculous disease, which characteristically destroys the disc space, partially destroys parts of two adjacent bodies which fuse on healing, and often involves another vertebral body.

Plate 4.9   AP view of the lumbar spine of an adult with a known carcinoma of the bronchus. Note that the spinous process of L3 is absent. This was due to a secondary deposit.

Periosteum

Normally the periosteum is not seen on an x-ray film. Its usual function is to maintain the cortex by laying new bone down in continuity with it, balancing the normal osteoclastic activity. However, a wide variety of stimuli may cause it to lay down new bone visible separately from the cortex, known as a periosteal reaction or periostitis. If such a reaction is seen, the three points to note are: (1) type of reaction; (2) distribution; and (3) associated lesions.

TYPE OF REACTION

Linear   A single linear shadow of bony density alongside the cortex, separated from it by a relatively transradiant line. This is commonly inflammatory, but may be the earliest stage of almost any type.

DISTRIBUTION

The most difficult task of all is the interpretation of a single isolated periosteal reaction on a single bone. It may be due to trauma – a healing fracture, a subperiosteal haematoma or the so-called traumatic periostitis. The two last-named conditions may only produce a localized fusiform thickening of the cortex. A linear periosteal reaction may be the only sign of a stress fracture, such as the 'march fracture' of the neck of a metatarsal. It may be due to infection; acute osteomyelitis is more likely to be towards the end of a long bone, usually associated with some soft-tissue oedema, and syphilis and yaws in the adult more commonly produce such a reaction on the shaft. A primary bone neoplasm (for example, osteosarcoma) is more common towards the end of a bone, especially the lower end of the femur, but a secondary neoplasm can appear anywhere in it and may produce a layered rather than a linear reaction.

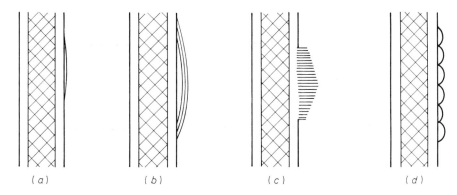

Figure 4.1   Diagram showing the common radiological appearances of periosteal reactions. (a) Linear –single layer. (b) Layered–so-called 'onion-skin' periostitis. (c) Spiculated–palisade. (d) Heaped-up.

Layered   Several layers of bony density parallel to the cortex (so-called 'onion-skin' periostitis); this is commonly malignant.

Spiculated   Fine spicules of bone point outwards from the surface of the bone, usually in groups or resembling palisades. These are usually malignant but can occur in infection.

Heaped up   An irregular wavy line of bone density lying alongside the cortex. This can be inflammatory but may also occur in some of the rarer metabolic conditions.

These various types of reaction are illustrated diagrammatically in *Figure 4.1*

Classically, a layered periosteal reaction in the shaft of a long bone is due to Ewing's tumour, a highly malignant primary lesion of youth. In many cases the subsequent progress of an initially undiagnosable linear periosteal reaction makes the diagnosis clear, either by resolving or showing additional signs.

If, however, there is more than one lesion, the distribution and type of reaction may give a clue. Widespread fine linear periosteal reactions are often seen on the long bones of immature infants, disappearing as growth proceeds. A somewhat similar appearance is seen in the idiopathic periosteal reaction of infants at a later age. A rather lumpy periostitis has been recorded in the phalanges and metatarsal bones in tuberose sclerosis, and is common in osteogenesis imperfecta due to healing of the numerous fractures. In the rare congenital melorheostosis, irregular dense new bone is laid down along one side of a long bone (often several bones in a limb). In infantile cortical hyperostosis (Caffey's disease), arising between the ages of 9 weeks and 5 months and usually resolving by the age of 12 months, there is a single linear periosteal reaction on any or many long bones, including the ribs, but it is often symmetrical and is commonest in the mandible and clavicles. There is often more separation from the cortex than in other conditions.

Multiple healing fractures at different ages in infants and children are seen in osteogenesis imperfecta and also in cases of non-accidental injury ('battered babies'); the former are distinguished by the thin cortex and sometimes excessive wormian bones in the skull, which allows differentiation from defective bone formation due to malnutrition associated with ill-treatment. Multiple fractures may also occur in old people. Fractures are more likely in osteoporosis, while the pseudo-fractures of osteomalacia should be recognized by involving one side of the cortex only with an associated periosteal reaction. These occur commonly in the anterior border of the scapula, the ribs, the pubic rami, the inside of the femoral neck or shaft, and the tibia or fibula.

Acute or subacute osteomyelitis in children is sometimes a generalized disease due to staphylococcal septicaemia, and more than one bone may be involved. This may also occur in salmonella osteitis in sickle-cell disease. Some chronic infections show periosteal reactions; they are rare in tuberculosis of bone but common in syphilis — linear in the congenital variety, usually symmetrical at the ends of long bones such as wrists, and often heaped and shaggy in the acquired variety, more commonly on the shaft of a long bone. Yaws is difficult to distinguish from syphilis.

In Reiter's syndrome, where the digits are involved in the arthritic process, linear periosteal reactions may be seen along the phalanges and sometimes along the metatarsals or metacarpals.

Secondary neoplasm may produce more than one lesion but they are commonly of different ages, and while one may show only a periosteal reaction another may show additional evidence of destruction.

Symmetrical periosteal reactions, either heaped or linear, on the extremities sometimes involving just the wrists and/or ankles, and in other cases extending from toes or fingers to knees or elbows, may be due to hypertrophic pulmonary osteo-arthropathy. This usually indicates lung carcinoma or other intrathoracic tumour, and is an indication for chest radiography.

A linear periosteal reaction occurs on the shafts of long bones in vitamin A poisoning, and is often also a feature of severe rickets. A heaped-up reaction is seen on the wrists in the condition known as thyroid acropachy (thyroid disorders associated with thickened skin) and also in the rare pachyderm-periostose which also has thickened skin. Scattered linear reactions may be seen in morphoea (beneath affected patches of skin), in xanthomatosis, and rarely in sarcoidosis.

ASSOCIATED LESIONS

Careful search must be made on the film for other signs which may assist in the diagnosis. Soft-tissue oedema is commonly due to infection, and though it is sometimes said that a very severe soft-tissue infection may produce an underlying periosteal reaction in a bone, infection of the bone is more likely. A chronic ulcer (for example, a varicose ulcer, a tropical ulcer, or one due to recurrent trauma on the shin) may have an underlying periosteal reaction. In advanced cases the bone may eventually become infected, and after many years malignant change may supervene in the ulcer with involvement of bone. Subperiosteal new bone is often found in association with arteriovenous and other vascular malformations, and when these form soft-tissue masses containing phleboliths the pattern is characteristic.

A thorough search should be made for fractures, especially in children. Periosteal new bone formation is a normal part of fracture repair but is not seen often in routine orthopaedic practice because it takes place during the time when the fracture is immobilized. Radiography is usually delayed until union seems likely. In child abuse, because of late reporting of the injuries, intermediate stages of repair can be seen, often not in the bone originally complained of; or a periosteal reaction on one bone may be explained by a fracture elsewhere.

Destructive changes in the infected bone occur in acute osteomyelitis. Initially, the medulla towards the end of the bone shows some faint rarefaction, which may precede the periosteal reaction in infants and younger children. Patchy destruction of the bone then proceeds, and a portion of cortex loses its blood supply. While the rest of the bone tends to become rarefied, this piece remains dense and is recognizable as a *sequestrum* of dead bone. Meanwhile, the periosteum lays down new bone surrounding the affected part, sometimes the whole bone, forming the *involucrum,* and holes in this through which pus can escape are known as *cloacae (see Figure 4.2).* A radiograph may be taken at any stage of this progression, and while only the earlier stages may

only, primary tumours of bone usually have simultaneous bone destruction and bone pro- duction (sometimes dense) in different parts. Occasionally, a solitary secondary lesion will mimic a primary. Sometimes the growing tumour

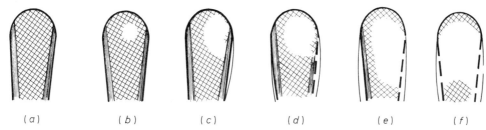

Figure 4.2   Diagram showing stages in the natural history of osteomyelitis. (a) Normal bone-end in a child. (b) Early trabecular destruction (may be minimal). (c) Trabecular destruction and periosteal reaction. (d) Increased periosteal reaction and cortical destruction. (e) Formation of sequestrum. (f) Subperiosteal new bone now forms an involucrum, enclosing the sequestrum, with a cloaca through which the pus may escape.

be seen where modern methods of diagnosis and treatment are available, later stages may be seen in developing countries. Other infections may also produce periosteal reactions; they occur along the affected bones in leprosy, and occasionally in sarcoid.

Destructive changes are a prominent feature of neoplastic lesions of bone. While a fine-layered

breaks through the periosteum, producing a characteristic sign; a triangle is formed by the remaining bony cortex. the elevated periosteum and the side of the advancing neoplastic mass (Codman's triangle)* *(see Figure 4.3).* Destructive changes in Ewing's tumour appear relatively late. The fine palisade appearance without destruction is rare but strongly suggestive of malignancy.

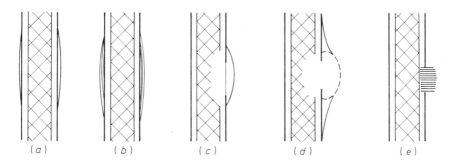

Figure 4.3   Diagram showing some periosteal reactions associated with malignant neoplasm. (a) Linear – single layer periosteal reaction, but often on both sides of the bone. (b) Layered – 'onion-skin' layering, usually Ewing's tumour or secondary malignancy. (c) Periosteal reaction with destruction of cortex and medulla. (d) Soft-tissue mass bursting through periosteum and raising it at the sides to form a triangle (Codman's triangle). (e) Palisade type of reaction – very fine bone spicules.

periosteal reaction may be the only initial sign, ill-defined loss of bone pattern soon appears in the underlying bone, followed by patchy or coalescent disappearance of bone altogether. There is no visible margin round the lesion. While secondary neoplasms are commonly destructive

A well-defined cystic lesion associated with a periosteal reaction may be a simple cyst with a fracture through it, or the rare benign chondro- blastoma of the upper end of the humerus; other- wise, benign tumours do not produce periosteal reactions. Histiocytosis X (eosinophil granuloma)

* Infection also occasionally does this.

also produces a cystic lesion which may have associated periosteal reaction.

In scurvy, the characteristic appearance is a massive subperiosteal haematoma, often associated with the rarefied appearance of the epiphysis and flattened dense metaphysis and sometimes with a metaphyseal fracture. Where a periosteal reaction is seen in rickets, the characteristic cup-shaped metaphysis is usually unmistakable.

The foregoing covers the commoner causes of periosteal reactions, but others may appear and some cases may be very difficult to solve. Some recognizable lesions are to be seen in *Plates 4.10–4.16.*

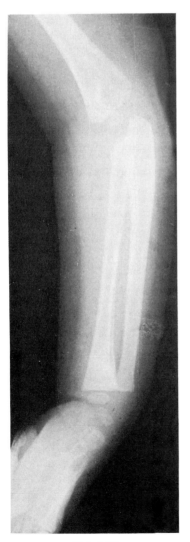

Plate 4.10

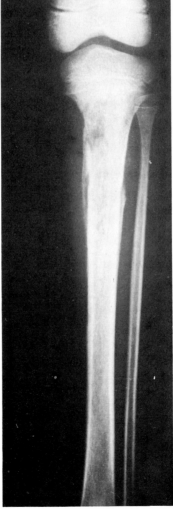

Plate 4.11

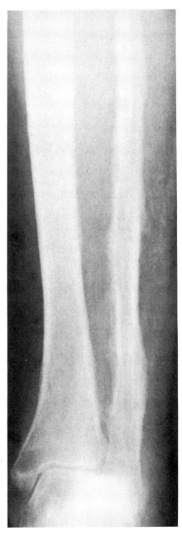

Plate 4.12

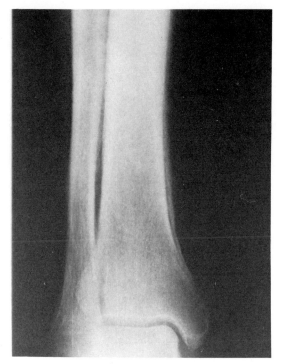

Plate 4.13

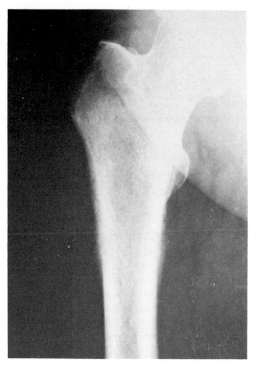

Plate 4.14

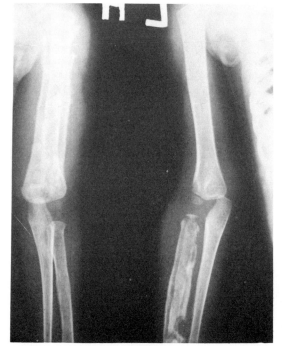

Plate 4.15

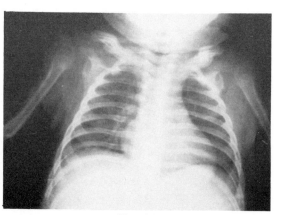

Plate 4.16

SOLUTIONS

Plate 4.10   Periosteal reaction on the ulnar side of the lower end of the radius, which is part of the process of healing of a greenstick fracture.

Plate 4.11   Periosteal reactions on both sides of the upper tibial shaft associated with destructive changes in the shaft and the formation of dense cortical sequestra – typical appearance of osteomyelitis.

Plate 4.12   Unusually extensive periosteal reaction on the fibula associated with a defect in the soft tissues due to a chronic varicose ulcer, to which the periostitis is a reaction.

Plate 4.13   Linear periosteal reaction running smoothly up the lower end of the tibia and fibula (better seen in the former). The smoothness and symmetry is against a local cause – this is the type of appearance produced by hypertrophic pulmonary osteoarthropathy, due to neoplasm of bronchus.

Plate 4.14   Layered periosteal reaction all round the upper shaft of the femur, with some loss of definition of the lateral cortex. Inflammatory disease is unusual at this site in an adult, though not impossible; malignant neoplasm is much more likely, either Ewing's tumour, or a secondary deposit. A primary osteogenic sarcoma is also possible but probably would show more evidence of bone production, and at this stage a more asymmetrical periosteal reaction. This was a secondary deposit from the gut.

Plate 4.15   Extensive periosteal reaction forming an involucrum in right humerus and left radius; in each bone the whole shaft has sequestrated and the involucrum has a cloaca for the discharge of pus. The diagnosis was typical chronic osteomyelitis in more than one bone.

Plate 4.16   Periosteal reactions on both clavicles, and also on the humerus on both sides, though less easy to see. These are typical sites and appearances of infantile cortical hyperostosis (Caffey's disease).

Cortex

CONTINUITY

The cortex should be traced right round the bone, starting at one corner of the supposed quadrilateral, and any discontinuity noted. These can be broadly grouped into breaks, defects and expansions. Care should be taken not to mistake normal anatomy, such as nutrient foramina, epiphyseal lines or fossae, for abnormalities.

Breaks   The commonest cause of a sharp discontinuity in the cortex is a fracture which may show a transradiant line or a step. Individual fractures are well described in other books but some principles are worth mentioning here.

While the whole fracture line may be shown across the bone, if displacement is slight only those fracture edges which lie in the plane of the x-ray beam will be visible (*Figure 4.4*). Examples are the spiral tibial fracture or a greenstick fracture in a child, fracture of the neck of the talus, and fracture of the neck of the femur in an old lady, in all of which the plane of the fracture is usually oblique to the beam. An alteration in alignment

may be the only sign. If Shenton's line in the hip (a smooth curve along the lower border of the femoral neck and the upper border of the obturator foramen) is lost then femoral neck fracture can be assumed, even without seeing the fracture edges. Many such assessments depend on symmetry. Incomplete fractures do occur, in osteomalacia (Looser's zones) and also in Paget's disease; stress fractures may be incomplete. A pathological fracture occurs through existing pathology, such as a bone cyst, a neoplasm or severe infection; unusual bone appearances near a fracture should be looked for.

Defects   By this is meant any depression or 'hole' in the bone. A defect at the end of a long bone may be due to joint disease, which will be discussed later. Elsewhere, a bony defect may be due to external pressure or erosion, an intrinsic lesion or endosteal pressure or erosion from a medullary lesion. Pressure may be from bands of fibrous tissue, other bony prominences, localized benign tumours (for example, neurofibroma) or aneurysm (for example, erosion of vertebral bodies by aortic aneurysm). Infections and neoplasms may involve bone by direct spread. The subperiosteal bone

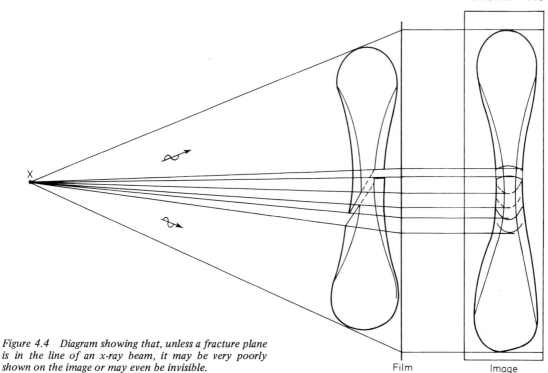

Figure 4.4   Diagram showing that, unless a fracture plane is in the line of an x-ray beam, it may be very poorly shown on the image or may even be invisible.

Film   Image

resorption of hyperparathyroidism is seen as small (less than 0.5 mm) almost semi-circular defects in the cortex of the middle phalanges, occasionally the toes. It is less noticeable in other bones but the tibia may have a more deeply concave upper medial border than usual.

Intrinsic cortical defects of infancy and childhood (Caffey's cortical defects) (for example, in the lower end of the femur) are of no clinical significance. Syphilis and yaws may produce small defects confined to the cortex, particularly in congenital disease and gummata, but periosteal reactions are common. Osteolytic neoplastic secondary deposits or primary bone tumours destroy bone *in situ* without altering the basic architecture and have ill-defined edges as they infiltrate. This distinguishes them from the much slower growing benign tumours with their well-defined edges and distortion of bone architecture. If the edges are better defined, though without a linear edge, they are more likely to be due to multiple myelomatosis (so-called 'punched-out' lesions) but distinction between this and secondary deposits may be impossible.

Endosteal defects may be due to benign cystic lesions within the medulla. A scalloped endosteal cortical edge is common in fibrous dysplasia.

Ill-defined endosteal cortical defects may be due to destructive medullary lesions such as infections (acute and chronic osteomyelitis, tuberculosis, syphilitic gumma) or malignant neoplasm (sarcoma, myeloma, secondary carcinoma).

Expansion   Expansion can take place in two ways: the whole cortex can be displaced outwards from the medulla, due to a slow-growing benign medullary lesion, usually being thinned in the process – this is the more usual meaning of the term; the cortex may also be expanded in both directions by an expanding lesion within it, again usually benign – the classical cause of this is the lobulated non-osteogenic fibroma with its internally scalloped edge. An osteoid osteoma has a similar effect but the cortex is more thickened than expanded with increase in bone density and a small central transradiancy, sometimes containing a tiny dense spot. A localized bone infection (Brodie's abscess) may have a similar appearance. A primary bone tumour (osteosarcoma) may by increasing bone production also appear to expand the cortex, but evidence of destruction and periosteal reaction is frequently present.

Plates 4.17–4.24 show some examples of cortical discontinuity.

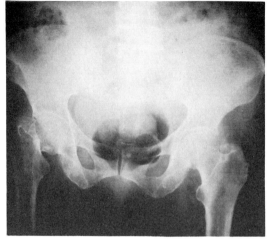

Plate 4.17

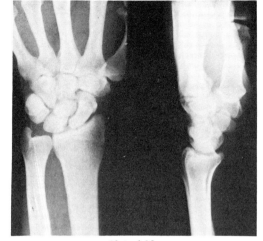

Plate 4.18

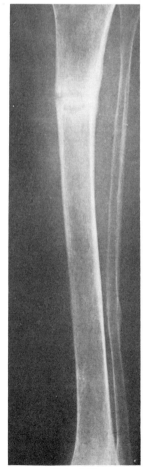

Plate 4.19

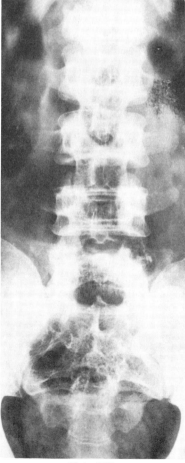

Plate 4.20

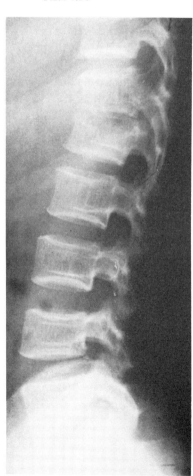

Plate 4.21

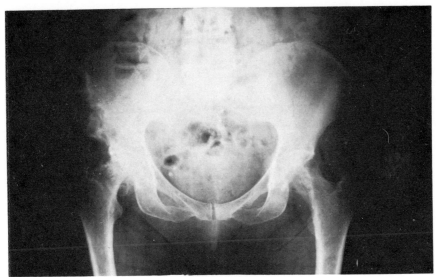

Plate 4.22

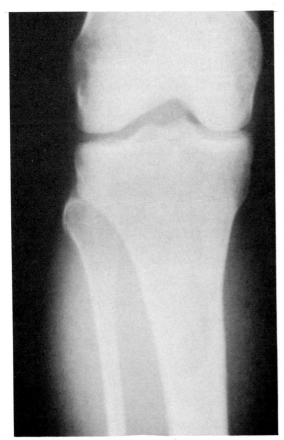

Plate 4.23

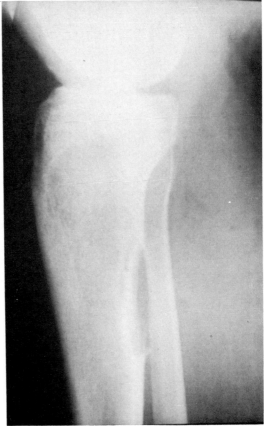

Plate 4.24

SOLUTIONS

Plate 4.17 AP view of the pelvis showing hip joints and upper femora. Note the smooth curve of the upper margin of the obturator foramen on the left continuing along the inferior surface of the femoral neck down on to the shaft; on the right this is disturbed and the femur is displaced upwards, due to a fracture of the neck of the femur. The fracture line itself is not readily visible and the diagnosis is inferred from the disturbance of the normal anatomical relationships.

Plate 4.18 AP and lateral views of the left wrist in a young adult; note that the radial epiphysis is virtually closed, only a trace remaining. This should not be mistaken for a fracture. Careful study of the carpal bones, however, shows that there are fractures of both the capitate bone and the scaphoid bone, a relatively unusual combination.

Plate 4.19 AP view of the left tibia and fibula in an adult. Note a relatively thin cortex and an incomplete fracture of the upper tibial shaft involving the medial part of the cortex only. Two fracture lines can be seen, corresponding to the anterior and posterior cortex. There is some associated cortical thickening indicating an attempt at repair. A similar but much less noticeable lesion is seen in the lower fibular shaft. These are typical Looser's zones or pseudo-fractures occurring in osteomalacia.

Plate 4.20 AP view of the lumbar spine. The body of L1 looks flatter than the others, and its upper border looks blurred, as does that of the adjacent lower border of T12. The lesion is almost off the picture, a not uncommon situation. (An artefact to the left of L2 should be ignored.)

Plate 4.21 Lateral view of the lumbar spine of the same patient as in Plate 4.20. It is now clear that the disc space at T12–L1 is obliterated, the upper border of the body of L1 has lost its clearly defined cortex, and there are destructive changes in the lower anterior part of the body of T12. These appearances are typical of chronic inflammatory disease, almost always tuberculous.

Plate 4.22 AP view of the pelvis, showing both hips. The disturbance of Shenton's line on the right indicates a fracture of the neck of the femur, but there are also several small defects in the neck of the left femur and an extensive irregular defect can be seen in the lateral part of the right ilium. The defects are due to osteolytic secondary deposits from a carcinoma of the breast, resulting in a pathological fracture of the right femoral neck.

Plate 4.23 AP view of the upper part of the right tibia and fibula. Note an oval defect in the tibial shaft.

Plate 4.24 Lateral view of the same case as in Plate 4.23. Note that there is expansion of the cortex both into and away from the medulla, an appearance virtually diagnostic of non-osteogenic fibroma.

THICKNESS

The cortex is normally at its thickest in the middle of the shaft of a long bone, and there are analogous differences in other bones. Changes in thickness may be generalized or localized as in all bone pathology. It is important to bear in mind the normal range of variation due to the quality of the radiography.

Increased cortical thickness   *Generalized* cortical thickening with increase in density is a characteristic feature of osteopetrosis (marble-bone or Albers—Schonberg disease), usually obvious at birth (in some unusual variants it may appear later). In other congenital bone diseases with relatively short bones (for example, achondroplasia, chondro-ectodermal dysplasia and related dystrophies) the cortex looks relatively thick, but in gargoylism (Hurler's syndrome) there is true thickening.

An adult with large hands and relatively thick cortices should be suspected of having acromegaly. Particularly well-formed solid-looking cortices would suggest hypoparathyroidism, a difficult diagnosis to make without biochemical evidence. Symmetrical calcification of the basal ganglia in the brain may occur.

In the rare congenital disease of melorheostosis, referred to earlier in the chapter, there are *localized* thickenings, and in progressive diaphyseal dysplasia (Engelmann's disease) there is a symmetrical fusiform cortical thickening of long bones, especially the tibiae. Cortical thickening may also be seen in fibrous dysplasia whether monostotic (one bone only) or polyostotic (involving several bones, usually asymmetrically), but cortical thinning is more common here due to expansion of the medulla. In haemoglobinopathies the cortex is thin in infancy and childhood but in later life it becomes thickened and in places wavy and irregular on the endosteal aspect.

Old fractures usually show some deformity and the thickened parts of the bone are relatively dense and smooth. More thickening is likely if there has been extensive remodelling to restore alignment, and in compound fractures and penetrating wounds (gunshot and the like). In children, fractures usually heal without trace. Multiple fractures may be due to multiple or repeated injury, non-accidental injury or osteogenesis imperfecta in children or osteoporosis or osteomalacia in adults.

Cortical thickening is common following inflammatory bone disease. In old chronic osteomyelitis, while the outside of the bone may be smooth there are often irregular well-defined internal defects, some due to bone destruction by the infective process, and others due to surgery varying from simple drilling to extensive guttering or sequestrectomy. Cloacae may persist. Dense sequestra may still be present. Old bone tuberculosis may look similar, away from a joint, but is usually less dense.

Tertiary syphilis may produce cortical thickening, especially over convex surfaces (for example, sabre tibia) but there is often also evidence of activity such as a periosteal reaction or medullary destruction due to gumma. Yaws produces a similar appearance. Congenital syphilis is more likely to show periosteal reactions and destructive changes in the metaphyses in the young but may produce thickening later on.

Extensive dense cortical thickening with fusiform expansion of the cortex is seen in the non-suppurative or sclerosing osteomyelitis (of Garré) presumed to be due to an organism of low virulence, without destruction or periosteal reaction; if more localized it can be due to bone abscess or osteoid osteoma, described above.

The cortex is often thickened in association with an angiomatous malformation, following the laying down of subperiosteal new bone.

Malignant neoplasm, particularly osteosarcoma, may in the early stages produce only a cortical thickening, sometimes dense, but periosteal reaction and/or destruction inevitably appear in a few weeks. While secondary neoplasm occasionally imitates this, it more often produces osteosclerotic or osteolytic lesions without disturbing the architecture.

The commonest cause of a thickened cortex in an older person is Paget's disease. Here the normal rate of bone resorption is increased and the new bone which replaces it is of reduced strength and of abnormal structure. It is a caricature of normal bone, as if amateurs had been at work, with thickened cortex, coarsened medullary trabeculae and lines of stress not in the normal places. Normal bone is laid down along the lines of stress, especially down lines of weight-bearing, so thickened cortex usually appears along the concavity of a shaft (for example, in bow-legs or knock-knees, or the remodelling of a fracture); but in Paget's disease, the cortical thickening is on the convex aspect of a bone as well as on the concave aspect. Syphilis and yaws also thicken the convexity but the general bony architecture is not disturbed as in Paget's disease.

Many of the conditions just described are due to increased subperiosteal new bone formation, and so may have shown a periosteal reaction in their earlier phases; and many periosteal reactions culminate as or pass through a stage of cortical thickening.

Cortical thinning The congenital condition of osteogenesis imperfecta (fragilitas ossium) has already been mentioned as a cause of multiple fractures, and its diagnostic feature is *generalized* cortical thinning. In the most severe cases, a still-born infant may have virtually every bone broken including ribs, preventing respiration. Various degrees of the condition exist up to that which only arises towards puberty (osteogenesis imperfecta tarda). As mentioned earlier, the distinction from malnutrition with ill-treatment may be difficult, but an excessive number of wormian bones in the skull can occur in osteogenesis imperfecta. In arachnodactyly (Marfan's syndrome) and homocystinuria the bones are long and slender and the cortex thinner than normal but not so fragile. Haemoglobinopathies (whether due to sickle-cell disease, thalassaemia, or related variants) and other severe congenital haemolytic anaemias are usually associated with a generalized increase in the amount of bone marrow to compensate for the increased rate of red cell destruction, so that the cortex may be markedly thinned and often expanded, particularly in the limbs and extremities in infancy and childhood. A somewhat similar effect occurs in Gaucher's disease in children, due to an increased lipoid storage in the marrow. Loss of femoral tubulation producing a club-shaped or 'hock-bottle' deformity may be seen in both these last two conditions.

A thin cortex in an adult is usually part of a generalized disease. It is difficult to find an unassailable term for this but 'generalized bony rarefaction' is probably the least misleading descriptive expression. The commonest is true osteoporosis, of which some degree is almost universal in post-menopausal women, worsening with age. Old men are not so badly affected. The bone is normal but there is not enough of it; blood biochemistry is normal though there is a small negative calcium balance. Not enough organic bone matrix is formed so that the normal rate of bone resorption has the advantage and replacement is slowed. The thinning of the cortex may not be obvious in the long bones, but in the vertebrae the appearance of the bodies is striking, especially in lateral view. Not only are the medullary trabeculae hardly seen, but the upper and lower cortex look as if they had been drawn with a fine hard draughtsman's pencil. Relatively minor accidents produce compression collapse of one or more vertebral bodies, and sometimes only the

pressure of the nucleus pulposus is required to induce a biconcave shape. In other bones fractures are easily acquired, notably the femoral neck and the lower end of the radius (Colles' fracture) in old ladies. Similar appearances are produced by artificial menopause in younger women and by other alterations of hormonal imbalance such as Cushing's syndrome (pituitary basophilism) and prolonged steroid therapy. Malnutrition may do the same but other evidence of dietary deficiency is likely.

Hyperparathyroidism may also show only a generalized bony rarefaction but careful scrutiny may reveal the phalangeal subperiosteal erosions, the granular appearance of the skull vault and loss of the lamina dura of the teeth, the altered trabecular pattern at the end of the long bones or even bone cysts. Hyperthyroidism also may be associated with generalized bony rarefaction, often concealed by the fact that the patient is thin anyway.

In osteomalacia, some cortical thinning may occur but it is not the diagnostic feature nor is it essential for the diagnosis; the appearance of the medullary trabeculae, general loss of bone density and the presence of Looser's zones (pseudofractures) are more important.

In all these conditions attempts have been made to quantify the extent of bone loss, and several methods have been devised in different centres. The most popular seems to be a metacarpal index which relates the thickness of the cortex at the centre of a metacarpal (usually third right) to the width of the bone. The student should acquaint himself with the method used locally.

Myelomatosis may present as a solitary myeloma (a single destructive lesion in one bone), multiple myelomata (widespread 'punched-out' bony erosions as well as soft-tissue lesions) or in the generalized form producing bony rarefaction. In the vertebral bodies the distinction of the latter from osteoporosis may be difficult, but myelomatosis tends to render the bodies more irregular in shape while the degree of cortical thinning is less than would be expected for the extent of the deformity.

In the congenital condition of fibrous dysplasia the increased amount of fibrous tissue in the medulla tends to produce *localized* endosteal thinning of the cortex, sometimes expanding it. Deformity may occur where normal bone is lacking along the lines of stress, as in the femoral neck. It may be monostotic or polyostotic, needing skeletal survey to find the various asymmetrical lesions.

Loss of cortical thickness in a distal part of a limb, sometimes most of it, may be due to disuse atrophy; common causes are trauma (fractures recently out of plaster), pain or hysterical paralysis. Organic sensory deprivation seems to have a specific trophic effect, for example, as in syringomyelia, toxic neuritis or peripheral nerve injury, and it produces a similar picture.

Inflammatory lesions may produce localized cortical thinning, initially due to the hyperaemia and later (as in osteomyelitis) by medullary destruction and expansion. The peri-articular bony rarefaction associated with inflammatory arthritis (for example, rheumatoid, tuberculous or septic) is a similar early sign.

The rare haemangioma of bone thins the cortex, ranging in appearance from the coarse trabeculation and thinned cortex of a single vertebral body, through the 'soap-bubble' expanding lesion to the extreme of the so-called 'vanishing bone disease'.

The cystic lesions of bone originating in the medulla all tend to expand and thin the overlying cortex, and it is important to decide where a cystic lesion arises.

Some examples of abnormalities of cortical thickness are to be found in *Plates 4.25 – 4.35*.

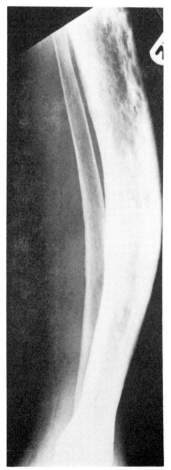

Plate 4.25

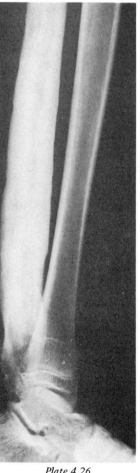

Plate 4.26

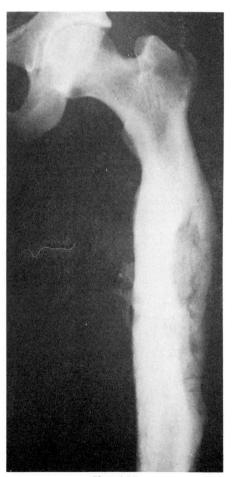

Plate 4.27

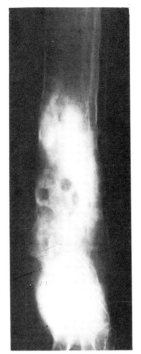
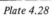

Plate 4.28

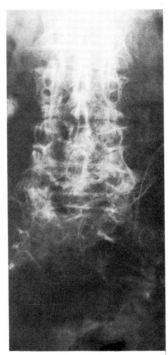

Plate 4.29(a)

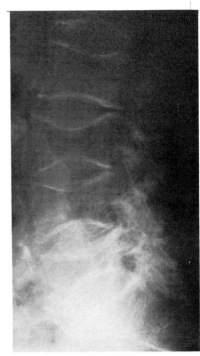

Plate 4.29(b)

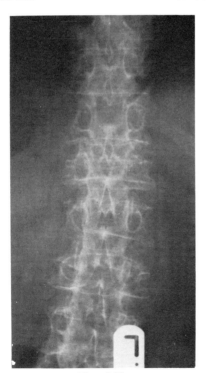

Plate 4.30

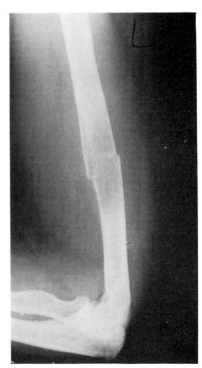

Plate 4.31

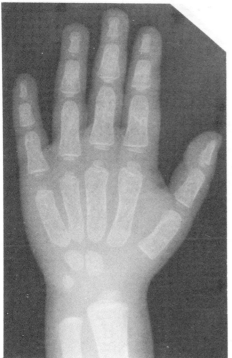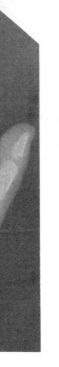

Plate 4.32

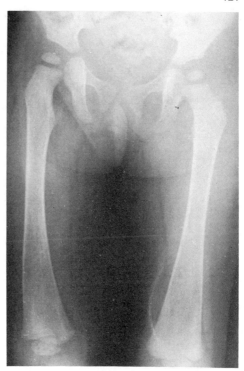

Plate 4.33

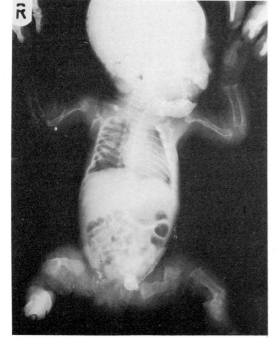

Plate 4.34

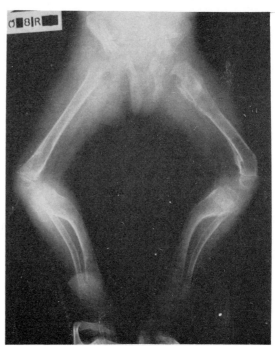

Plate 4.35

SOLUTIONS

Plate 4.25   Lateral view of right tibia and fibula. Both anterior and posterior cortices are thickened and the medulla also shows some coarsening of its trabeculation. The tibia is bowed convex anteriorly and there is cortical thickening along the convexity. Appearances are typical of Paget's disease.

Plate 4.26   Lateral view of the left tibia in an older child. Marked cortical thickening of the fibula, the tibia being normal. This was due to yaws in an African girl.

Plate 4.27   AP view of the left femur and hip showing dense cortical thickening in the medial cortex of the shaft with some new bone formation. There has also been some thickening of the lateral cortex but there is an extensive defect. This is most likely to be due to surgery – 'guttering' – of a very severe old osteomyelitis, following a compound fracture.

Plate 4.28   AP view of the tibia, fibula and ankle on the left. The bone is grossly widened and densely thickened in its lower third, being rarefied with a thin cortex and an old periosteal reaction above this. There are numerous defects in the lower part and the ankle joint has been destroyed. This could only be due to long-standing chronic infection; in this case it was actinomycosis, the so-called 'Madura foot'.

Plate 4.29   (a) AP view of the lumbar spine and sacrum, showing considerable bony rarefaction with thinning of the cortex; osteoarthritic changes are also present. (b) Lateral view of the lumbar spine of the same case; note the thin upper and lower cortices of the vertebral bodies, very little visible bone trabeculation in the medulla of the bodies, and partial collapse of the centres of the bodies. This is osteoporosis.

Plate 4.30   AP view of the lumbar spine. Note the thin cortex and the generalized rather irregular flattening of the vertebral bodies. It would be difficult to distinguish this from the osteoporosis shown in Plate 4.29(b) except for the variability between affected bodies. This was myelomatosis.

Plate 4.31   Lateral view of the left humerus, showing expansion and thinning of the cortex in the centre of the shaft with a fracture through it. The edges of the lesion are ill-defined where it meets normal bone and there is clearly bony destruction in the middle of the bone. This is a pathological fracture through a secondary deposit from carcinoma of the breast.

Plate 4.32   The hand and wrist of a child showing a thin cortex everywhere and poor medullary trabeculae; the cortex is somewhat expanded so that the metacarpals and phalanges are almost oblong. This is characteristic of a haemoglobinopathy, but in this case it was thalassaemia.

Plate 4.33   The femora of a child showing loss of tubulation and modelling of the lower shafts which are said to resemble a hock bottle in shape; there is some cortical thinning. This appearance is usually described in association with Gaucher's disease, due to the lipoid storage in the bone marrow, but in this case it was due to a haemoglobinopathy (sickle-cell disease, homozygous SS).

Plate 4.34   AP view of a baby showing a thin cortex everywhere and numerous fractures in long bones and ribs. Notice the umbilical cord, indicating the first few days of life. This is the typical appearance of osteogenesis imperfecta (fragilitas ossium) at birth.

Plate 4.35   AP view of both legs of a child showing gross deformity. The pelvis is compressed from side to side. There is periosteal new bone formation on the left femur and both tibiae, though less extensive. The tibiae are bowed, convex medially with a rotation deformity also. The clue to the aetiology is the very thin cortex, permitting the diagnosis of osteogenesis imperfecta, and the deformities are due to malunited fractures. It should be noted that on the concavities of the deformed tibiae the cortex is slightly thicker, showing that even defective bone tends to be laid down along the lines of weight-bearing.

DENSITY

It may be difficult to assess bone density when there are variations in cortical thickness but comparison with normal bone, either elsewhere in the body or in another patient should help. Changes in bone density indicate abnormality of bone formation rather than of structure.

Increased bone density (bone sclerosis) The four classical causes of *generalized* bone sclerosis are osteopetrosis (Albers—Schonberg or marble-bone disease), fluorosis (due to the ingestion of excessive fluoride in areas where the water has a high fluoride content), secondary carcinomatosis and Hodgkin's disease. Osteopetrosis is distinguished by the somewhat club-shaped bone ends and the thick cortex in the middle of the shafts, and in fluorosis the sites of musculo-tendinous attachments show exaggerated bony prominence. The two neoplasms may show increase in density without change in shape of the bones. Some generalized increase in bone density also occurs in renal osteodystrophy.

Where the increase in bone density is widespread rather than generalized, often asymmetrical, there are several possibilities which are usually recognizable by the pattern of the abnormality. The congenital conditions of osteopoikilosis (collections of dense spots in long bones near joints, but not in the skull) and osteopathia striata (linear streaks running towards the ends of long bones) are characteristic. Probably of similar nature is the occasional dense bone island near a joint. Widespread patches, spots or nodules of bone sclerosis without alteration of the basic shape of the bone are likely to be due to secondary carcinoma, commonly from the prostate gland in men, but it can be from any of the common neoplasms, for example, breast, thyroid, bronchus. Usually the axial skeleton is most heavily involved, the extremities rarely and late. In Paget's disease there is often widespread increase in bone density but some asymmetry is inevitable and the typical caricature of bone architecture with a thickened cortex is usually recognizable.

Localized bone sclerosis is present in many of the conditions with a thickened cortex already described, notably localized Paget's disease, old injuries and infections, and it is also sometimes an early sign of an osteosarcoma. A single patch of sclerosis may be a metastasis. The common causes of a single dense vertebral body are Paget's disease (usually with some enlargement), Hodgkin's disease (not usually so dense, sometimes with a periosteal reaction and/or ligamentous calcification) and secondary carcinoma (no change in size). An apparent increase in density may be seen where the liver overlies a lower thoracic vertebra in lateral view. A triangular dense shadow, sometimes associated with low back pain in parous women, lying on the lateral side of the sacro-iliac joint, is known as osteitis condensans ilii. It is not usually regarded as of clinical significance.

Decreased bone density Very few conditions produce true generalized decrease in bone density. Virtually all the various conditions producing generalized bony rarefaction have normal bone but there is not enough of it. In osteomalacia and rickets, however, in which lack of vitamin D or its analogues or metabolites prevents the conversion of osteoid to bone, there is enough bone (sometimes more than usual in osteomalacia) but it is of poor quality.

Probably the commonest cause of localized loss of bone density is neoplastic infiltration of large or small areas, the edges of which are ill-defined.

In the conditions producing cortical thinning the remaining bone is normal. In the so-called fibrous variety of Paget's disease, the abnormal bone pattern is seen but with a loss of density instead of an increase.

Some examples of alterations in bone density are given in *Plates 4.36—4.39*; in some the radiography has been adjusted to show the bone detail, and the bone texture must be taken rather than the 'whiteness' alone. These *Plates* should be studied systematically because in at least two this permits a firm diagnosis.

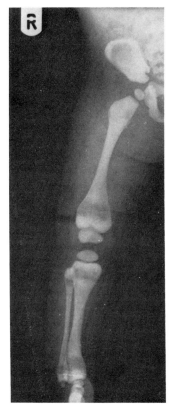

Plate 4.36

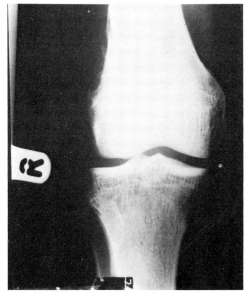

Plate 4.37(a)

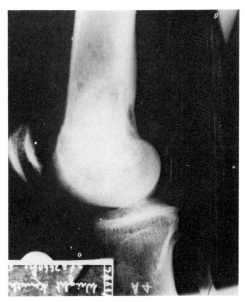

Plate 4.37(b)

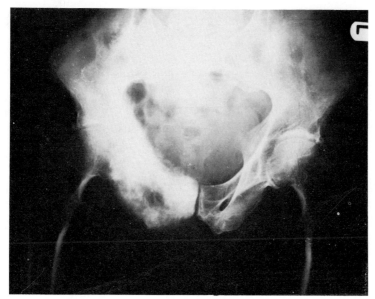

Plate 4.38

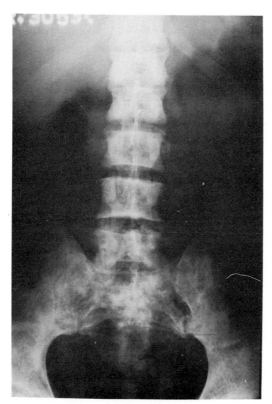

Plate 4.39

SOLUTIONS

Plate 4.36   AP view of the leg of a child. The cortex is thick and very dense, particularly in the metaphyses, with transradiant regions beneath these. The ends of the bones are widened. The increased density has to some extent been reduced by increasing the radiographic factors, but with normal factors this would be very dense indeed and much of the detail shown here would be invisible. The appearances are typical of osteopetrosis (Albers–Schonberg or marble-bone disease).

Plate 4.37   (a) AP view of the right knee showing a dense area in the lower end of the femur, with evidence of destruction in the lateral cortex. This combination is strongly suggestive of an osteogenic sarcoma. (b) Lateral view of the same knee. The dense region in the centre of the bone is again shown.

Plate 4.38   AP view of the pelvis, showing increased density of the right side, particularly in the ischium and pubis. The normal bone texture has been replaced by a rather irregular, almost woolly-looking, material, which would do for Paget's disease; but in addition careful scrutiny of the medial border of the right pelvic brim shows a palisade type of periosteal reaction, typical of malignant disease. This is sarcoma occurring in Paget's disease of bone.

Plate 4.39   AP view of the lumbar spine and pelvis, showing scattered dense lesions, almost certainly due to secondary deposits. The primary was in the prostate gland.

Medulla

Again, three factors should be noted concerning the medulla and fitted into the picture already built up from studying the periosteum and the cortex: they are (1) the trabecular pattern; (2) any defects within it; and (3) any medullary calcification.

TRABECULAE

A generally coarse trabecular pattern is seen in haemoglobinopathies, as a consequence of the more extensive marrow, most obvious in infants and children. It may also be seen in the very rare fibrogenesis imperfecta, with scattered denser patches.

Generalized thinning and loss of trabeculae occurs in osteoporosis, myelomatosis and Gaucher's disease. In hyperparathyroidism the generalized loss of density in the medulla is seen on close scrutiny to be due to trabecular thinning, but there are more trabeculae in a very fine network, particularly seen near the end of a long bone. This fits with the concept of increased osteoclasis with normal bone replacement; where osteoclasis gets the upper hand completely, cystic defects appear (osteitis fibrosa cystica).

In osteomalacia, persistence of the osteoid seam means the bone is less dense and is also less rapidly reabsorbed since osteoclasts normally only remove normally calcified bone. The trabeculae are thus thicker and coarser but less dense than usual, giving rise to a characteristic 'woolly' appearance. If Looser's zones are also present, a firm diagnosis is possible. Where this state of affairs persists, the low blood calcium stimulates parathyroid activity, and the features of secondary hyperparathyroidism are added to those of osteomalacia; subperiosteal erosions, more Looser's zones, possibly cystic medullary changes and a characteristic appearance in the vertebral bodies, an increased density in the upper and lower thirds. This is the so-called 'rugger-jersey' spine, with horizontal stripes.

In fibrous dysplasia, the trabeculae are replaced with fibrous tissue. This may resemble 'ground glass', the trabeculae may be coarse and thick on a dense background, and calcification may occur. The cortex may be normal but is more often thinned from within and sometimes expanded. Rarely, the whole bone may be enlarged and dense. Whether monostotic or polyostotic, asymmetry is the rule.

Sarcoid produces an irregular dense coarse condensation of the trabeculae with some weakening of the cortex which may expand or collapse.

A generally thickened and dense trabecular pattern is seen in myelosclerosis (or myelofibrosis) associated with a leuko-erythroblastic anaemia.

DEFECTS

Defects in the medullary pattern may be difficult to assess, but the location, the nature of the edge and the presence of other abnormal signs are of help. Inflammatory lesions (osteomyelitis or tuberculosis), simple cysts and primary bone tumours are more likely near the end of a long bone. An ill-defined edge may be seen in the early stages of an osteomyelitis and is almost always a significant feature of malignant neoplasm, which destroys and replaces the bony trabeculae without displacing them. The neoplasm is usually more extensive than appears, and more than half of a vertebral body has to be affected before the lesion is seen radiographically. Primary bone tumours usually show new bone production as well as destruction but are rare, while secondary neoplasm is common and usually destructive, occasionally sclerotic and, rarely, productive.

A defined edge to a defect without a true rim is seen in multiple myeloma but there are usually numerous small lesions. A single lesion like this near the end of a bone may be an osteoclastoma, and in the shaft an eosinophil granuloma (histiocytosis X). Near a joint (for example, above the acetabulum) the pseudo-tumour of haemophilia is a rare but dangerous condition since biopsy without anti-haemophilic precautions may be fatal.

If the defect has a clear, well-defined edge, virtually a thin cortical margin, this means that the lesion has grown sufficiently slowly to allow the surrounding bone to be compressed and to 'wall-off' the lesion. It is thus almost certainly benign. A simple bone cyst at the end of a bone is the commonest, and the bone cysts of hyperparathyroidism are similar. Bone tuberculosis in children can also look like this particularly the disseminated type. Chronic osteomyelitis of low virulence may produce a similar bony reaction (Brodie's abscess) varying from a thin rim indistinguishable from the other causes to a very thick mass with a relatively transradiant centre similar to an osteoid osteoma. Hydatid cyst of bone is rare but tends to occur in the shaft. Several benign bone tumours have well-corticated edges, including aneurysmal bone cyst, chondroma and benign chondroblastoma. Cartilage tumours often contain calcification, and the rare chondroblastoma, near an epiphysis, is virtually the only benign tumour to have an associated periosteal reaction. The pseudo-cysts of osteoarthritis, if large, occasionally mimic other lesions.

Associated signs to look for are involvement of the cortex in any destructive process, as in neoplasm, and periosteal reactions which occur in both infection and neoplasm.

This is a very large subject which has only been briefly surveyed here. The diagnosis is clearly fraught with difficulty. If the student can distinguish between a benign and a malignant lesion, and inflammatory disease of bone, he will be doing very well indeed.

Vertebral body collapse   A medullary lesion of a vertebral body may lead to collapse, partial or complete, which may obscure the characteristic signs of the lesion. Disorder of ossification may mimic this, for example, a butterfly vertebra (two separated ossific centres), or a hemi-vertebra (one centre on one side only), but the bone looks otherwise normal and fusion or other anomalies of the appendages will be seen. Compression fractures produce anterior or lateral wedging and a clear angulation of the vertical cortex most compressed. This angulation becomes rounded off on healing.

Inflammatory disease produces slow partial collapse. If tuberculous, usually two or more adjacent bodies are involved with destruction of the intervening disc and a paravertebral abscess which may contain calcification. The bodies eventually fuse. Less extensive changes occur with other infections, for example, staphylococcal, but the distinction can be difficult.

Secondary neoplasm is a well-known cause and may be difficult to distinguish from myeloma.

A single flattened vertebral body in a child (Calve's disease, vertebral plana once thought to be due to osteochondritis and then eosinophil granuloma) may follow almost any such lesion, but unsuspected or undisclosed trauma is probably the commonest cause. True osteochondritis of the epiphyseal plates (Scheuermann's disease) produces flattened vertebral bodies with narrowed irregular disc spaces but not true collapse.

Multiple vertebral body collapse occurs in osteoporosis, osteogenesis imperfecta (multiple compression fractures), secondary neoplasm and multiple myeloma.

CALCIFICATION

This may be seen in fibrous dysplasia, chondroma and chondrosarcoma, and helps to identify the lesions. A solitary calcification at the end of a long bone may be the bone infarct of caisson disease (in those who work in high air pressures).

Plates 4.40–4.49 illustrate some medullary lesions. Use of the systematic scrutiny will allow a firm diagnosis in several, but in others it will only be possible to place the lesion in a class, for example, benign, malignant, congenital, inflammatory.

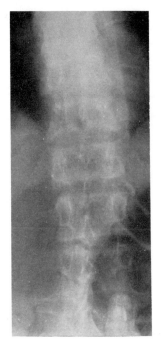

Plate 4.40(a)

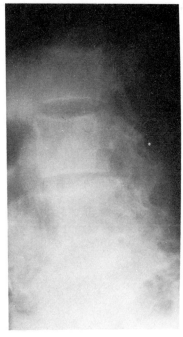

Plate 4.40(b)

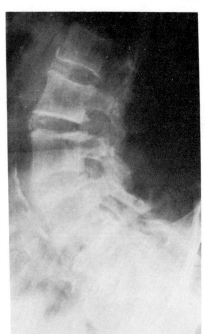

Plate 4.41

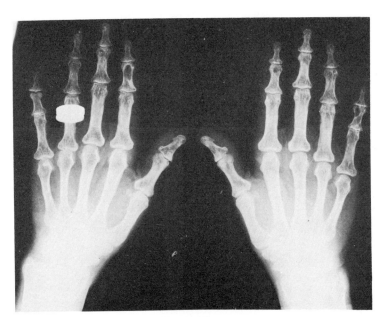

Plate 4.42(a)

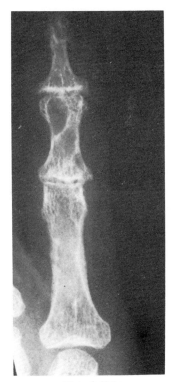

Plate 4.42(b)

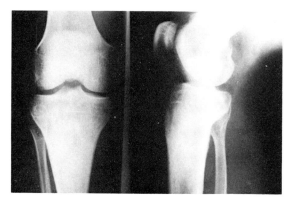

Plate 4.43

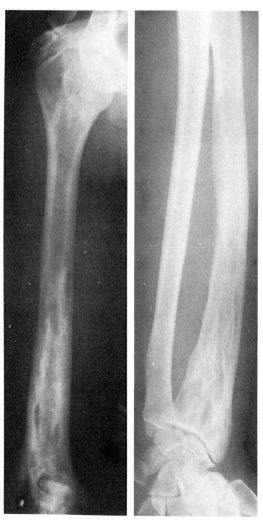

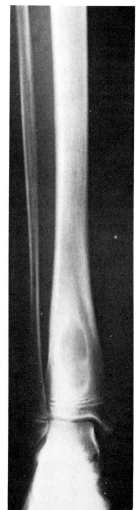

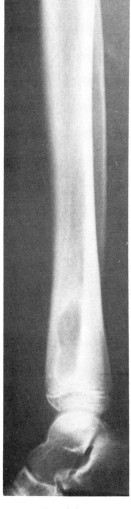

Plate 4.44(a)   *Plate 4.44(b)*   *Plate 4.45(a)*   *Plate 4.45(b)*

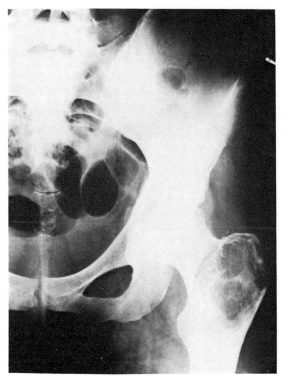

Plate 4.46

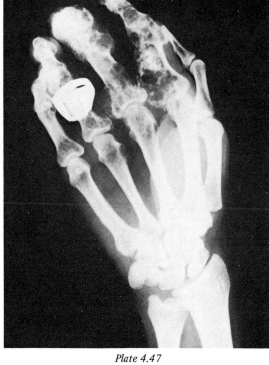

Plate 4.47

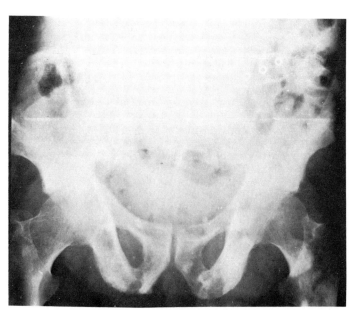

Plate 4.48

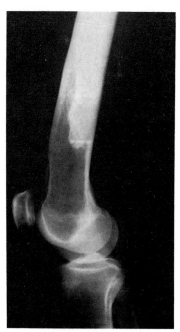

Plate 4.49

SOLUTIONS

Plate 4.40   (a) AP view of the lumbar spine. All the bony structures show a rather ill-defined, almost 'woolly' or 'fluffy' appearance, and the cortex is virtually of normal thickness. This is typical of fully fledged osteomalacia. (b) Lateral view of the same lumbar spine. Note the normal thickness of the cortex but poorly defined medullary trabeculation in the vertebral bodies. In comparison with the osteoporosis shown in Plate 4.29(a) and (b) the contrast between cortex and medulla is much less marked.

Plate 4.41   Lateral view of the lumbar spine. Note the normal thickness of the cortex, and the relatively increased density of the medullary trabeculae in the upper and lower thirds of each vertebral body, the middle third being relatively transradiant. This occurs in osteomalacia associated with hyperparathyroidism, often due to renal disease. (It is often known colloquially as 'rugger-jersey' spine, from the tradition of English Rugby players to wear jerseys with horizontal stripes.)

Plate 4.42   (a) Both hands of a woman with hyperparathyroidism. There are several cysts in the medulla, and careful scrutiny of the cortex of the phalangeal shafts will reveal subperiosteal resorption; this is present in the radial borders of the proximal phalanges of both little fingers and the middle phalanges of the right middle and ring fingers. (b) Enlargement of the right little finger of the same patient showing the cystic changes and the subperiosteal resorption.

Plate 4.43   AP and lateral views of the right tibia and fibula, showing a central rounded defect in the upper tibial shaft which is slightly expanded. The defect is relatively well-defined and the bone round it is rather sclerotic. The location is a common site of bone infection and the sclerotic bony reaction is in favour of this also. It was a Brodie's abscess, containing pus.

Plate 4.44   (a) AP view of the humerus showing alteration of the marrow trabeculation with some cortical thickening. (b) AP view of the forearm of the same case, showing alteration of the medullary trabeculation into irregular longitudinal strands with some thinning of the cortex. This appearance, and that of the humerus, are two variants of fibrous dysplasia.

Plate 4.45   (a) AP view of left tibia and fibula showing a bilocular cystic defect in the lower end of the tibia. The lesion is surrounded by a rim of dense bone but there is not much else in the way of bony reaction. (b) A lateral view confirms that the cystic lesion is central in the medulla and, again, bony reaction is confined to the edges of the lesion. This proved to be a simple cyst.

Plate 4.46   AP view of left hip, showing a cystic lesion expanding the greater trochanter of the femur. It has trabeculae separating it into locula. The appearances are typical of an osteoclastoma.

Plate 4.47   Left hand showing numerous cystic lesions expanding the phalanges of the index, ring and middle fingers. In places there are calcifications; the appearances are typical of multiple enchondromata.

Plate 4.48   AP view of the pelvis showing numerous small transradiancies, of varying sizes, reasonably but not sharply defined. Typical appearances of secondary deposits, in this case from carcinoma of breast.

Plate 4.49   Extensive calcification in the medullary cavity of the left femur (seen in lateral view) of a man who undertook deep-sea diving under high air pressures. Typical appearance of the bone infarct associated with this type of occupation.

JOINTS

Joints are more complicated than just the junction of bone ends. Soft tissues are even more important because some are part of the joint, the bone ends themselves deserve a careful look, and the bone ends in childhood can be most informative. The suggested sequence is shown in *Table 4.2*

Some joint diseases tend to involve specific joints. The distribution therefore, may be of help. Osteoarthritis can involve any joint but the common sites are the cervical and lumbar spines, distal interphalangeal joints of the fingers, the hips and the knees. Rheumatoid arthritis usually involves

seen in tuberculous arthritis, associated later with calcification. Soft-tissue swelling may also occur with gout, including the tophi (collections of urate crystals) but these may be away from the joints.

JOINT CAPSULE

It is helpful to know the extent of the capsule in each joint. In the fingers and toes they fit the joints closely, so the synovial granuloma (pannus) of rheumatoid arthritis produces early erosions. In other larger joints they are normally much more

Table 4.2

SCRUTINY OF JOINTS

I Soft tissues	II Bone ends	III Bone ends in childhood
(1) Peri-articular tissues	(1) Subarticular cortex	(1) Epiphysis
(2) Joint capsule and ligaments	(2) Joint margins	(2) Epiphyseal line
(3) Joint space	(3) Medulla	(3) Metaphysis

the proximal interphalangeal and metacarpo-phalangeal joints of the fingers, the wrists, some-times the toes, and knees and occasionally the hips and the cervical spine. Psoriatic arthritis tends to involve both interphalangeal finger joints; Reiter's disease involves the sacro-iliac joints, the toes and the fingers. Tuberculous infection is more likely in the spine, but the wrist, the hip and the knee are perhaps commoner sites than the other joints. Ankylosing spondylitis is normally con-fined to the spine and sacro-iliac joints, but there is a variety in which large joint involvement predominates.

Soft tissues

PERI-ARTICULAR TISSUES

Broadly speaking, joint diseases are of two kinds — those with an inflammatory type of lesion and those with degenerative disorder. Most of the former show peri-articular swelling at some stage, seen on the radiograph not only by thickening but also by loss of the dark lines between the joint and the skin normally produced by fat in the fascia separating muscles, ligaments, tendons and other structures. These are obscured by oedema. This appearance may be seen in rheuma-toid arthritis round proximal interphalangeal joints, the wrist or the knee joint. It is most marked round an acute suppurative arthritis and is also

extensive and become even more so when distended by an effusion. The soft-tissue shadow of a knee joint effusion may be seen, for example, in the supra-patellar pouch, or behind the joint. Elsewhere, a swollen capsule may be revealed by displace-ment of other structures, such as the transradiant supratrochlear pads of fat above the elbow joint pushed clear of the bone by the effusion, and the lateral displacement of the muscle bundles around the hip joint. Joint effusions occur in joint injuries (when it is most important to exclude fractures) and in most types of arthritis, commonest in the inflammatory types.

Loose bodies in joints may disappear into unlikely joint recesses. They may be due to osteo-chondritis dissecans, fractures, separated osteo-phytes (especially in neuropathic joints), pieces of synovial granuloma (melon-seed bodies), or the osteochondromatous bodies of synovial chondro-matosis. They have to be distinguished from other opacities, calcifications and sesamoid bones of which the fabella, in the tendon of popliteus behind and lateral to the lateral femoral condyle, is a good example.

JOINT SPACE

This is the space between the subarticular cortex of the adjacent bone ends. Normally filled by articular cartilage with only a film of joint fluid separating the two layers, it is increased when an effusion is present, and decreased with loss of cartilage. Thus, in inflammatory joint disease there is usually an increase in joint space at first. It may revert to normal but if there is cartilage damage it will be decreased later. This is common in septic arthritis and in tuberculous joint disease. In rheumatoid arthritis, the erosion is marginal to begin with and the joint space preserved until the damage is extensive or subluxation occurs. In degenerative joint disease such as osteoarthritis, either primary or secondary to joint damage, the initial lesion is loss of cartilage so loss of joint space is an important early sign.

Assessment of joint space is difficult unless the opposite side is normal for comparison and in children even more so because the epiphysis is wholly or partly of cartilage which is non-opaque.

Calcification of articular cartilage occurs occasionally, in the rare metabolic disease of ochronosis (alcaptonuria), in haemosiderosis, in hyperparathyroidism and other causes of hypercalcaemia, and in the condition of 'pseudo-gout' (chondrocalcinosis) in which calcium pyrophosphate crystals appear in the joint fluid in the elderly.

Bone ends

SUBARTICULAR CORTEX

Inflammatory joint disease produces bony rarefaction round the joint. In acute conditions, such as a suppurative arthritis, some of the bone looks as if it had been partly erased, as from a pencil drawing. If the bone is not involved, it may return to normal but residual bone defects are more likely. The 'rubbed out' appearance is also seen in tuberculous arthritis but it appears more slowly and is often followed by blurring of the joint surfaces. In rheumatoid arthritis, peri-articular rarefaction occurs early, followed by marginal erosions, the centre being preserved until late. Such a joint is unstable and subluxation occurs easily. Psoriatic arthritis and Reiter's syndrome behave similarly but the distribution is different.

In degenerative joint disease such as osteoarthritis, cartilage loss produces more stress on the subarticular cortex which becomes eburnated — thickened and polished — shown radiologically by thickening and increased density in the regions of greatest pressure. This is often along the line of weight-bearing, for example, in the knee joint the greatest changes are seen in the medial compartment of a bow-legged person and vice versa.

Secondary osteoarthritic changes occur in any deranged joint due to injury or disease and may be seen superimposed on, for example, old rheumatoid disease.

Gross abnormality of subarticular cortex is seen in neuropathic disease with sensory impairment from any cause (for example, tabes dorsalis, syringomyelia, diabetic neuropathy, peripheral neuritis or nerve injury, or congenital indifference to pain). Minor injuries are made worse by continued use of the joint, and ununited fractures, subluxations, malalignments, separated loose bone fragments and dense thickening of the bone ends should suggest this diagnosis.

JOINT MARGINS

Normally the subarticular cortex joins the shaft in a smoothly rounded corner. In rheumatoid arthritis, the synovial granuloma tends to erode the margin from the side of the joint, beginning with a small area of localized rarefaction. In gout, the urate deposit in the bone produces a defect near the margin which enlarges, may expand the shaft and eventually break through the joint margin. In typical cases, the point of origin of the defect is clear but the distinction can be difficult, and histiocytosis X (eosinophil granuloma) may resemble either condition. The flattening of the joint surfaces in osteoarthritis means that the margins are constantly abrading each other; the reaction is to lay down more dense bone growing outwards in the form of osteophytes. This is exaggerated in the neuropathic joint, and the osteophytes often fracture and fall into the joint.

ADJACENT MEDULLA

The medulla near a joint shows any rarefaction, and will be the site of infection where it extends into the bone from the joint. In osteoarthritis, cystic appearances (known as 'pseudocysts') are common. They are distinguished from the erosions of rheumatoid arthritis and the defects of gout by being larger with denser outlines in the presence of a dense intact, often thicker, subarticular cortex. In old rheumatoid disease, small cysts are common, some due to the secondary osteoarthritis and others due to burrowing into the bone by the pannus.

Figure 4.5 shows diagrammatically the radiological appearances in the fingers of some common joint diseases.

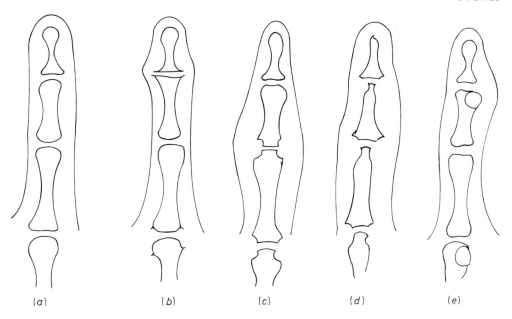

Figure 4.5   Diagram illustrating the different types of joint x-ray appearances produced by (a) normal, (b) osteoarthritis, (c) rheumatoid arthritis, (d) psoriatic arthritis and (e) gout as they can appear in a finger.

Joints of the spine and axial skeleton

Only the apophyseal and cervival neurocentral joints are simple diarthrodial joints. The sterno-clavicular joints have an articular disc between two compartments. The sacro-iliac joints and the pubic symphysis are synchondroses and the vertebral bodies are joined by ligaments and the intervertebral discs. Soft-tissue shadows may be seen round inflamed sterno-clavicular joints, Paraspinal masses are most commonly cold abscesses due to tuberculous infection of the vertebral bodies (particularly if calcified) but may be seen with other infections, with malignant disease, or histiocytosis X (eosinophil granuloma). Inter-vertebral disc generation may produce sclerosis and osteophyte formation in adjacent bodies (loosely termed osteoarthritis), seen also in old osteochondritis (Scheuermann's disease). True osteoarthritic changes occur in the apophyseal and neurocentral joints, especially if there are changes in alignment. Rheumatoid disease can occur in these joints, and in those between the atlas and axis vertebra; the destructive pannus may dissect between intervertebral disc and bone, so that partial collapse and subluxation can occur — very dangerous in the cervical region. Progressive ligamentous ossification in spinal joints associated with blurring, irregularity and eventual obliteration of the sacro-iliac joints, is characteristic of ankylosing spondylitis. Initially, the vertebral bodies look 'squared-off', progressing to the 'bamboo spine' appearance, best seen in the thoraco-lumbar region. In childhood and adolescence the normal sacro-iliac joints are wide with poorly defined margins, which should not be mistaken for pathology.

In the rare conditions of ochronosis, the inter-vertebral discs are flattened and dense.

Plates 4.50–4.62 show some typical examples of joint disease.

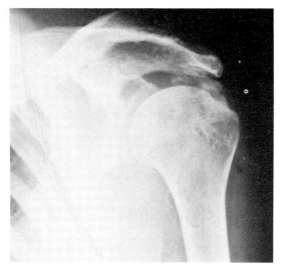

Plate 4.50

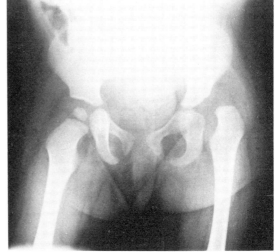

Plate 4.51

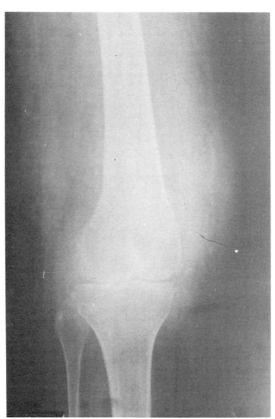

Plate 4.52

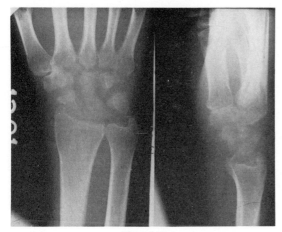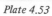

Plate 4.53

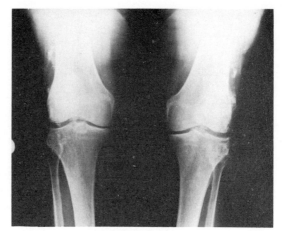

Plate 4.54

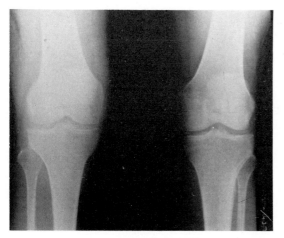

Plate 4.55

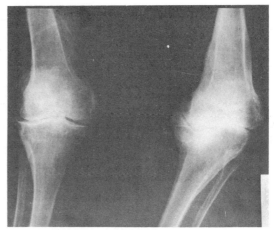

Plate 4.56

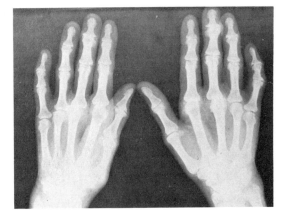

Plate 4.57

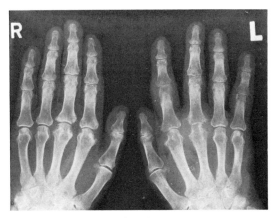

Plate 4.58

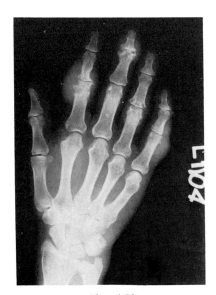

Plate 4.59

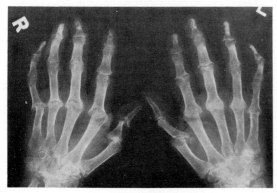

Plate 4.60

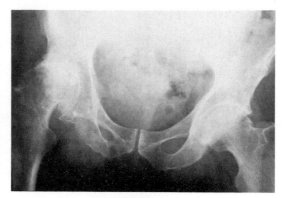

Plate 4.61

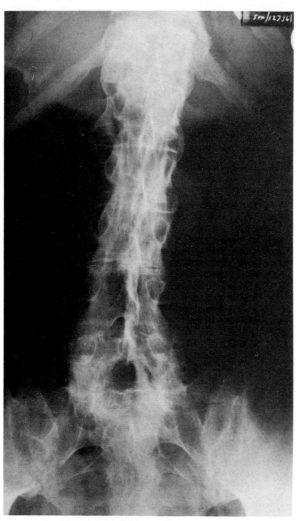

Plate 4.62

SOLUTIONS

Plate 4.50 AP view of a left shoulder, showing calcification in the region of the supraspinatus tendon, usually referred to as supraspinous tendinitis.

Plate 4.51 AP view of a child's pelvis; the right hip is normal but on the left the femoral capital epiphysis has not yet developed, the femur is displaced upwards and the roof of the acetabulum slopes upwards at a greater angle than on the right (40 degrees compared with the normal 23 degrees). This is congenital dislocation of the left hip.

Plate 4.52 AP view of a right knee, showing very marked soft-tissue oedema with marginal erosions at the medial edge of the joint. This is a suppurative arthritis.

Plate 4.53 AP and lateral view of a left wrist showing bony rarefaction and loss of definition of the cortex of most of the carpal bones, and the adjacent bone ends of the radius and metacarpals. This is due to tuberculous infection.

Plate 4.54 AP view of both knees showing joint space narrowing in both medial compartments with only slight osteophytosis but several loose bodies, particularly extending up into the suprapatellar pouch; one variant of osteoarthritis.

Plate 4.55 AP view of both knees showing calcification of the cartilage; this is chondrocalcinosis or 'pseudo-gout'.

Plate 4.56 AP view of both knees showing marked joint-space narrowing and sclerosis with subluxation. There are also periosteal reactions up both femoral and left tibial shafts, and on the left the joint is grossly disorganized with medial subluxation and angulation of the tibia. This is a neuropathic joint, in this case due to tabes dorsalis (Charcot's joint).

Plate 4.57 Dorsi-plantar view of both hands. Joint space narrowing and osteophytosis is most marked in the distal interphalangeal joints, although several of the other joints are also involved. This is typically osteoarthritis.

Plate 4.58 There is some peri-articular bony rarefaction in both hands, particularly in the proximal interphalangeal joints which also are surrounded by soft-tissue swelling, and there are marginal erosions, most extensive in the metacarpo-phalangeal joints. Appearances are typical of rheumatoid arthritis.

Plate 4.59 Left hand showing subarticular bony defects associated with localized soft-tissue swellings. This is typical of true gout, with both urate deposits in the bones and tophi in the soft tissues.

Plate 4.60 Dorsi-plantar view of both hands. Very severe destructive changes can be seen in most of the small joints and the anatomy of the carpus is barely recognizable. This is an advanced stage of rheumatoid arthritis.

Plate 4.61 AP view of the pelvis showing a normal left hip joint but considerable deformity of the right hip. There is joint space narrowing, sclerosis, compression of adjacent bone surfaces, pseudocyst formation and osteophytosis — all typical of advanced osteoarthritis.

Plate 4.62 AP view of the lumbar spine. There is a moderate scoliosis concave to the left. Although the disc spaces can be seen, in the upper part the intervertebral ligaments are calcified to produce the 'bamboo spine' appearance, nowhere can the apophyseal joints be seen clearly, the spinous processes seem to be part of one continuous structure (due to ossification of the interspinous ligaments) and the sacro-iliac joints are obliterated. This is typical of ankylosing spondylitis.

Bone ends in childhood

The bone ends during growth can be useful indicators of both general and local disease. If normal, they can be used to assess age, by reference to published books or charts, and the progress of some diseases may be estimated by the skeletal age. Normally, the knee-joint epiphyses and the ossific centres for talus, calcaneum (and often cuboid) are present at birth, and the femoral capital epiphysis at one year (not necessarily symmetrical). Other centres appear at intervals, and most fuse soon after puberty except for the iliac crest and the inferior angle of the scapula which are often visible after 20 years. Surprisingly, the epiphysis for the medial end of the clavicle does not appear until the age of 20 years and fuses after about one year. Skeletal maturation is retarded in hypothyroidism, hypopituitarism and related endocrinopathies, diabetes, coeliac disease, congenital heart disease, haemolytic anaemias, severe malnutrition and recurrent infections. Acceleration is rarer but may occur in hypergonadism and other endocrinopathies leading to precocious puberty, in excessive obesity and mongolism.

Abnormal bone ends may show characteristic appearances, but often it is only possible to place an individual case in a broad group of congenital, traumatic, inflammatory, neoplastic or metabolic lesions. The epiphysis, the epiphyseal line and the metaphysis should be looked at in turn, although the characteristic patterns usually involve all three.

EPIPHYSES

The epiphyses are irregular in a number of congenital bone diseases, sometimes calcified, and there are usually some associated deformities of the metaphyses. They are always well defined and the bone is otherwise normal. They are occasionally displaced by injury, though the 'slipped epiphysis' of the upper end of the femur may have other causes. Sclerosis and fragmentation of an epiphysis or ossific centre may be traumatic but is usually called osteochondritis. Some sites are common and all have eponyms, for example, upper femur (Perthé), vertebral epiphyseal plates (Scheuermann), tibial tubercle (Osgood—Schlatter), carpal lunate (Kienbock) tarsal scaphoid (Kohler), and head of second or third metacarpal (Freiberg).

Osteochondritis may be difficult to distinguish from aseptic necrosis due to injury or infarct (as in haemoglobinopathy).

A very rarefied epiphysis with a thin cortical rim occurs in scurvy, and a dense one with a thick rim is a feature of idiopathic hypercalcaemia. Tuberculous epiphysitis may be cavitated.

EPIPHYSEAL LINE

This is normally the transradiant space between the epiphysis and the metaphysis, wide in the very young, narrowing as the child grows and finally disappearing when fusion occurs. It is widened in rickets and hypophosphatasia.

METAPHYSIS

Irregular though well-defined metaphyses are seen in the congenital metaphyseal dystosis and unusual shapes in some other congenital conditions. Fracture or displacement of the metaphysis may be accidental but is also a feature of non-accidental injury as in 'battered babies', especially involving the wrists and knees. Periosteal reaction will be seen if the radiograph is delayed. Increased density and thickening of the metaphysis is seen in lead poisoning (lead line) and may also be produced by bismuth, phosphorus and vitamin D overdosage. It may also occur in congenital syphilis, but is usually associated with a transradiant zone beneath it and with periosteal reactions.

A thick dense band a little way from the metaphysis is seen in idiopathic hypercalcaemia, thicker than the lead line, and in the pelvis and vertebra, this gives the 'bone within a bone' appearance. In scurvy the metaphysis is dense but thin with a thin transradiant zone beneath it, and there are often fractures at the edges ('corner sign'). Large associated subperiosteal haematomata are common.

A single broad transradiancy in several long bones, a little away from the metaphysis is seen in leukaemia (for example, in both humeri on a chest film) indicating secondary deposits (usually symmetrical).

A blurred thickened metaphysis is a distinctive feature of rickets, because the conversion of osteoid to normal bone is delayed in the absence of vitamin D. Subperiosteal new bone, because its osteoid layer is much thinner, is delayed less (though a linear periosteal reaction may be seen), so as growth proceeds more bone appears at the edges of the epiphyseal line than at the metaphysis. This produces a cup-shaped metaphysis with a wider epiphyseal line. Because it is less stable, as

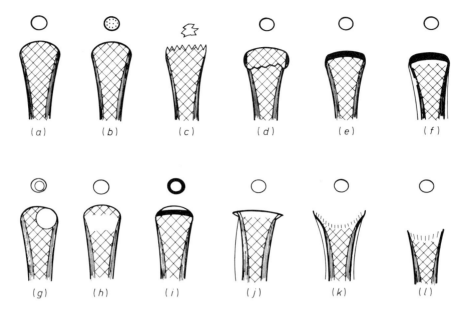

Figure 4.6   Diagrams illustrating some disorders of the bone ends in childhood. It is emphasized that these are cartoon figures and exaggerate the features which may appear more subtle in the radiograph; and they will differ in the extent to which they will be recognizable in different bones and at different ages. (a) Normal. (b) Chondrodysplasia calcificans congenita (epiphysis calcified). (c) Metaphyseal dysostosis (irregular metaphysis). (d) Metaphyseal fracture (with periosteal reaction; displacement may be minimal). (e) Lead poisoning (dense metaphyseal line). (f) Congenital syphilis (dense metaphyseal line but with transradiant line beneath it, and periosteal reaction). (g) Tuberculous infection (cavities can occur in both metaphysis and epiphysis). (h) Leukemia (transradiant zone a little way from the metaphysis). (i) Idiopathic hypercalcaemia (dense line a little way from the metaphysis, and thickened outline of epiphysis). (j) Scurvy (dense metaphyseal line, but thin and projecting with a transradiant zone beneath it. Thinned outline of epiphysis. May have subperiosteal haemorrhages also). (k) Rickets (cup-shaped metaphysis with poorly defined, slightly thickened metaphyseal line, farther from the epiphysis). (l) Hypophosphatasia (poorly defined metaphyseal line, well separated from the epiphysis.

the infant becomes more mobile so the margins of the 'cup' are forced outwards. The degree of abnormality depends on the severity, varying from mild nutritional rickets to severe metabolic disease due to failure to absorb or use vitamin D, for example in coeliac or renal disease, or even due to drugs such as phenytoin.

Some typical appearances are diagrammatically illustrated in *Figure 4.6* and some examples can be seen in *Plates 4.63–4.71*.

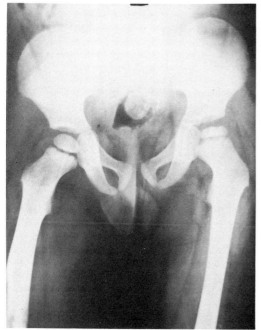

Plate 4.63

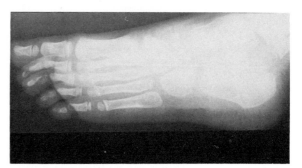

Plate 4.64

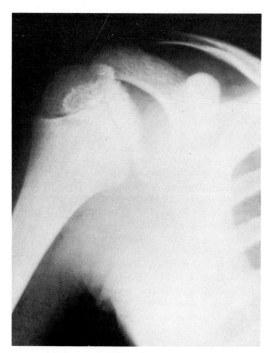

Plate 4.65

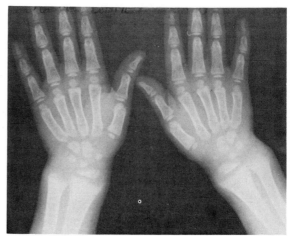

Plate 4.66

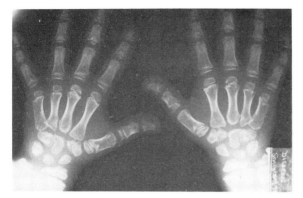

Plate 4.67

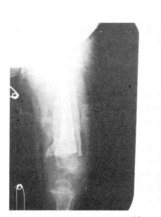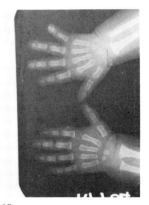

Plate 4.68

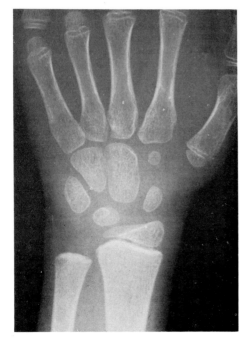

Plate 4.69

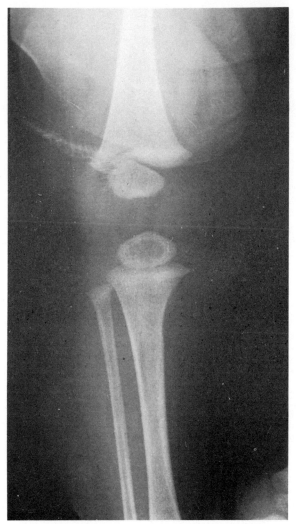

Plate 4.70

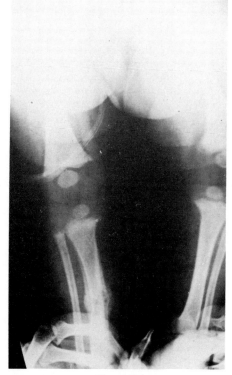

Plate 4.71

SOLUTIONS

Plate 4.63 *AP view of both hips, showing increased density and flattening of the left femoral capital epiphysis. This is typical of osteochondritis, usually referred to as Perthe's disease.*

Plate 4.64 *Oblique view of a child's foot, showing flattening of the scaphoid bone. This is typical of osteochondritis, usually known as Kohler's disease.*

Plate 4.65 *AP view of the right shoulder showing increased density with irregularity and flattening of the epiphysis for the head. This might have been regarded as an osteochondritis were it not for the fact that it occurred in a patient with a haemoglobinopathy (sickle-cell disease) and is most likely to be due to aseptic necrosis following infarction.*

Plate 4.66 *Forearms and wrists of a child. The bones all look slightly rarefied. The ends of the radius and ulna show a cup-shaped deformity and some expansion, typical of rickets, but the space between the metaphysis and the radial epiphysis is now partly filled with irregular bone and there is some sclerosis round the region. This suggests that this is healing rickets, and the subperiosteal new bone is part of the healing process.*

Plate 4.67 *Both hands and wrists of a child, showing considerable irregularity of metaphyses and epiphyses. This can only be due to a congenital bone disease; in this case, the chondro-osteodystrophy of Morquio and Brailsford.*

Plate 4.68 *Dorsi-plantar views of both hands and wrists and a lateral view of the knee joint of a child. The metaphyses of the long bones show a narrow band at the end with a narrow transradiant band beneath it, and, in addition, the femur shows subperiosteal new bone being laid down a considerable way from the shaft, presumably on a subperiosteal haematoma. The tibia shows some general rarefaction with a relatively thin cortex and the knee epiphyses also look rarefied with a 'pencil-thin' cortex round them. This is typical of scurvy.*

Plate 4.69 *PA view of the wrist of a child, showing a narrow dense band at the metaphysis of both the radius and the ulna. There is no transradiant band beneath it and the bones look otherwise normal. This is characteristic of lead poisoning.*

Plate 4.70 *AP view of knee joint in a child. The metaphysis shows in both femur and tibia a thick and rather ill-defined dense band and the epiphysis also has a thickened dense cortex round it. This was a case of idiopathic hypercalcaemia, and the differences from scurvy and lead poisoning can be seen.*

Plate 4.71 *AP view of both knees of a young child, although the left is only partially shown. There is a healing fracture of the right tibia, with callus and a periosteal reaction, but this is not all. There are transradiancies through the callus on the medial side of the fracture, indicating refracture, suggesting that it has not been immobilized, and there is also evidence of another, more recent, fracture on the medial side of the right femoral metaphysis. This suggests non-accidental injuries on several occasions. In addition, the tibial metaphyses are wider and less sharp than usual, suggesting some degree of rickets. This radiograph thus raises the possibility of a social problem which may not have been obvious clinically.*

| # The Skull

Radiography of the skull may be undertaken either for suspected local injury or disease of the bones of the skull, or for suspected intracranial disease. These may be quite separate or inextricably interrelated.

The anatomy is complicated, and though every student has in his time known it well enough, its elucidation on radiographs tends to be the province of the specialist radiologist. Views in several directions are required to show the anatomy fully, and these fall into three groups: lateral views, the x-ray beam being perpendicular to the sagittal plane; antero-posterior (AP); or posterior-anterior (PA) views with the x-ray beam in the sagittal plane, and various special oblique views. The student is advised to base the study of the skull on the lateral view, using the other views only to check certain points as they arise. Most correctly positioned lateral views look alike but views with the x-ray beam in the sagittal plane are liable to some variation in spite of attempts at international standardization. The five common views of this type are illustrated in *Figure 5.1*. There is nothing easy about either the radiography or the interpretation of these projections, and larger works may be consulted for more anatomical detail and the precise angles involved.

The following scheme of scrutiny of the skull therefore applies to the lateral view of the skull. Other views will be mentioned later as necessary.

GENERAL SIZE AND SHAPE

Estimates of the age from the skull are difficult but unerupted teeth are seen in the smaller skulls of children and usually only older adults are

Table 5.1

SCRUTINY OF THE SKULL

(1) General size and shape	(5) Pituitary fossa
	Size
(2) Scalp and soft tissues	Defects
	Shape
(3) Vault	
Markings	(6) Intracranial calcifications
Normal	Normal
Abnormal	Abnormal
Defects	
Normal	(7) Facial region
Abnormal	Sinuses
Thickness	Upper facial bones
Increased	Mandible
Decreased	Airway
(4) Base	(8) Cervical spine
Shape	
Fossae	
Temporal bone	

edentulous. Obvious deviations from expected size and shape should be noted, such as increase in the size of the vault, usually due to hydrocephalus, or reduction in size (microcephaly), and unusual shapes due perhaps to craniostenosis (premature closure of one or more sutures). Slight asymmetry is common and of no significance, but more marked degrees may be due to cerebral hemiatrophy on the smaller side or old subdural haematoma, cyst or tumour on the expanded side — more likely arising in childhood when the skull is still growing and thus malleable. In general

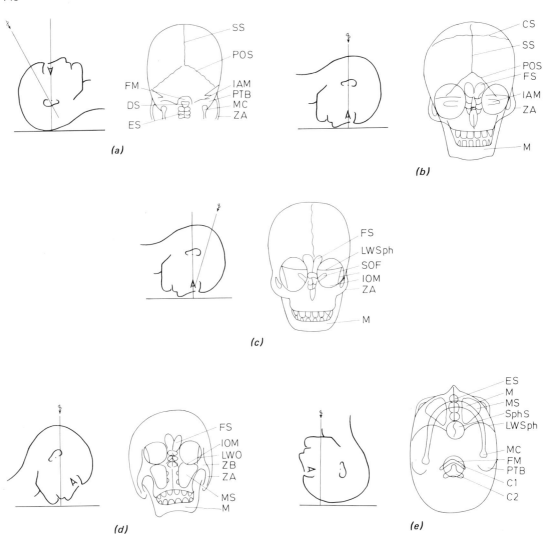

Figure 5.1 Diagram showing the principal anatomical features demonstrated in the common views of the skull taken with the x-ray beam in the sagittal plane. The exact angles of tilt are not given here since they vary in different centres and different reference lines may be used. (a) Towne's view (fronto-occipital with tube tilt to the feet). (b) Postero-anterior or occipito-frontal view. (c) Postero-anterior or occipito-frontal view with tube tilt to the feet. (d) Occipito-mental view. (e) Submento-vertical or basal view.

SS–Sagittal suture	ZA–Zygomatic arch	IOM–Inferior orbital margin
POS–Parieto-occipital suture	MC–Mandibular condyles	LWO–Lateral wall of orbit
CS–Coronal suture	FS–Frontal sinus	MS–Maxillary sinus (antrum)
FM–Foramen magnum	ES–Ethmoid sinus	ZB–Zygomatic (malar) bone
DS–Dorsum sellae	M–Mandible	SphS–Sphenoid sinus
PTB–Petrous temporal bone	LWSph–Lesser wing of sphenoid	C1–Atlas vertebra
IAM–Internal auditory meatus	SOF–Superior orbital fissure	C2–Axis vertebra

Other structures are, of course, visible, but those illustrated and indicated are those which the projections show best. It should be added that a good basal view also shows most of the basal foramina and even detail of the middle and inner ear, but these are very much the province of the specialist radiologist.

the sight of a skull which looks unusual in shape should lead to further investigation, usually starting with reference to radiological textbooks.

SCALP AND SOFT TISSUES

Soft tissues of the skull often look even darker than in other bone x-ray films, but by passing the film over a strong light in circular fashion it is possible to detect skin tumours, sebaceous cysts, bony prominences or unusual dense shadows due to metal or glass fragments in the scalp which might otherwise be regarded as intracranial. Modern vehicle windscreen glass fragments have a characteristic irregular quadrilateral shape.

VAULT

The vault of the skull normally shows its inner and outer tables separated by the diploë but there is a wide range of normal variation in thickness both absolutely and relative to the diploë which is occasionally virtually obliterated.

Markings

NORMAL MARKINGS

The following are the normal markings to be looked for.

Sutures   In lateral views the coronal and parieto-occipital sutures should be easily visible (though the parieto-temporal may be less so because of the oblique apposition of its edges); the sagittal, parieto-occipital and occipito-temporal sutures should be visible in Towne's view. They are wider in infancy, become narrower and more zig-zag in childhood, and in the adult end-up as well-defined but irregular linear transradiancies. They are fixed in position, so that their appearance is predictable from the way in which the film has been taken. It is most important to be sure that the film has been taken 'straight', that is, with the skull correctly aligned, since a slightly 'off-lateral' or rotated PA or Towne's view will make the sutures look asymmetrical or unanatomical and one of them may be mistaken for a fracture.

Vascular markings   In the majority of lateral views the groove for the middle meningeal artery can be seen in the squamous temporal bone, dividing into its anterior and posterior branches. It can be

distinguished from other linear shadows by being smooth, regular and straight or arching, and, when dividing, doing so at angles of about 45 degrees. These grooves on the two sides may be super-imposed, or separated so that the lines look doubled. The venous channels through the diploë are much more irregular and it is usually impossible to see any sort of drainage pattern, although there is often a large channel running laterally and downwards close behind the coronal suture. In general, venous channels are wider than the arterial chennels, and much more irregular in course and calibre; often, one or the other pre-dominates in a particular skull. It is possible to see fine corticated edges in nearly all vascular markings.

Dural venous sinuses   Where the edge of the dura is attached to the bone a ridge is raised — a parallel pair for each sinus. These are not normally visible on lateral views but in Towne's view the torcula herophili or confluence of the superior sagittal, lateral and straight sinuses can be seen; there is usually some asymmetry. Occasionally the sigmoid sinuses are well shown.

ABNORMAL MARKINGS

Sutures   The sutures themselves may be obliterated in the various forms of craniostenosis. They may be pulled apart (diastasis) in raised intracranial tension in children; the normal zig-zag appearance becomes blurred as four edges appear — one for each table in each bone. When well marked the appearance is characteristic, but lesser degrees may not be demonstrable. An excessive number of wormian bones is seen in two conditions — cleido-cranial dystosis and osteogenesis imperfecta.

Fractures   Most fractures are not difficult to recognize. Linear fractures tend to remain the same width and do not branch in any regular fashion; they cross vascular markings, and they may cross suture lines, but often there is a change in course or the suture itself may be involved in the damage. Sometimes, because of different lines of breakage in the two tables, the edges do not remain parallel but appear to narrow and widen in places. Scratches on the film may cause confusion but can be eliminated by viewing it obliquely by reflected light.

Care should be taken to note whether a fracture appears to run into the frontal sinuses or the petrous temporal bones or mastoids, permitting connection with the exterior and therefore becoming a variety of compound fracture. A depressed fracture may be difficult to see unless the x-ray beam is tangential to the skull. It may be only shown by an ill-defined slightly denser semi-circle where the overlapped edges make a double shadow at one side of the depression. Extensive fractures in young children may show a coarse mosaic or 'crazy-paving' appearance, which suggests considerable force and leads to suspicion of non-accidental injury. The suture or fracture on the side nearest the film will appear sharper, and for this reason in some centres both lateral views are taken in traumatic cases. A Towne's view and a PA view with downward tilt of the x-ray beam (or equivalent AP view) show the occipital and frontal bones respectively and the Towne's view also shows the petrous temporal bones.

Abnormal vascular markings   The venous channels are normally so irregular that increased vascularity of the skull may be difficult to recognize, but it does occur in association with meningioma and sometimes vascular malformations.

Defects

NORMAL

Pacchionian granulations produce rounded transradiancies in the inner table, usually within 2 cm of the sagittal sinus — they are normal. Smaller transradiancies, 1–2 mm in diameter, may be apertures for emissary veins.

ABNORMAL

Abnormal defects should be assessed by their size, position, shape, the nature of their edges and whether single or multiple. A single well-defined small defect, if mid-line, may be due to meningocoele or dermoid cyst. Other small well-defined defects may be difficult though usually benign. A haemangioma is crossed by irregular lines, dermoid and epidermoid cysts expand, eosinophilic granuloma may have a scalloped edge, and a dense centre may be seen in fibrous dysplasia. Penetrating injuries, burr-holes, craniotomy flaps and other surgical defects are usually obvious. Irregular defects may be due to radiation necrosis or to osteomyelitis — coccal, tuberculous or syphilitic. If the edges are poorly defined, neoplasm is likely, either due to local spread or metastasis.

Multiple small defects can occur in haemoglobinopathy. Multiple 'punched-out' rounded defects of varying sizes, well-defined but without corticated edges, are usually due to myeloma, which may also involve the mandible (which is generally spared by metastases). Multiple small defects occur in Letterer–Siwe disease in infants (a lipoid storage disease).

Extensive well-defined defects occur in another lipoid storage disease, Hand–Schuller–Christian disease ('geographical skull') in younger patients and in osteoporosis circumscripta of Paget's disease, in older people. Here, large areas show rarefaction with a sharply defined edge, usually asymmetrical ignoring sutures and involving frontal and/or occipital bones. Involved areas may be separated by normal bone but dense 'woolly' thickening of the outer table, typical of Paget's disease, may be present elsewhere in the vault.

Thickness

INCREASE

Increased thickness is usually associated with an increase in density; the two commonest causes are hyperostosis frontalis interna, an irregular thickening of the inner table of the frontal bone, not uncommon in middle-aged women and of no clinical significance, and Paget's disease. In the latter, the thickening is confined to the outer table (again the convex aspect of the bone) and is usually of a 'woolly' or 'fluffy' nature with ill-defined 'lumps' of dense material mixed with less dense material. This appearance should not be mistaken for sclerotic secondary deposits, which are rare and occur in normal bone without distortion of its architecture. Other causes of thickening of the skull vault are less common; sometimes the external occipital protuberance is unduly prominent and can easily be seen in a lateral view but forms an odd-looking density in Towne's view.

In severe forms of haemoglobinopathy (usually sickle-cell disease (SS) or thalassaemia) one of the ways of supporting the additional bone marrow is for additional bone to be formed in the outer table of the skull in the form of radiating spicules — the typical 'hair-on-end' appearance.

Osteopetrosis, although principally involving the base, can also produce an increased thickness and density in the vault, especially in the adult, and fibrous dysplasia can do the same in a more localized manner. Ivory osteomata are easily recognized. A relatively rare but important lesion is the dense local thickening in association with a meningioma, at first principally involving the inner table — meningiomatous hyperostosis.

DECREASE

Some thinning occurs in severe hydrocephalus; in the congenital condition of craniolacuna the whole vault consists of boneless patches separated by bony bands of normal thickness. Occasionally there is bilateral thinning of both parietal bones. Expansion of the vault with very thin bone may be seen over a subtemporal decompression operation site. The vault is poorly developed in cleido-cranial dysostosis and osteogenesis imperfecta.

Some examples of normal and abnormal appearances of the vault of the skull are to be found in *Plates 5.1–5.9,* but scrutiny should start with a general look at the size and shape and at the scalp and soft tissues.

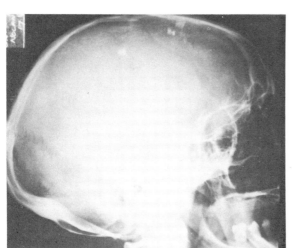

Plate 5.1

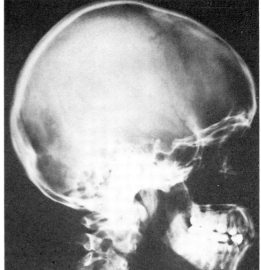

Plate 5.2

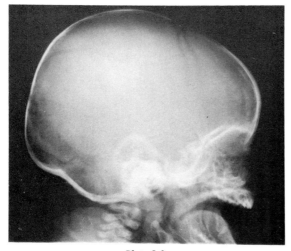

Plate 5.3

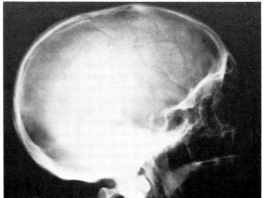

Plate 5.4

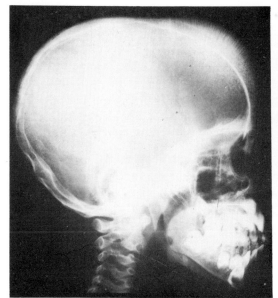

Plate 5.5

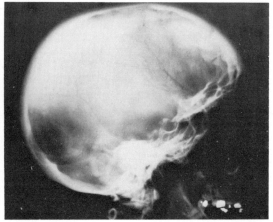

Plate 5.6

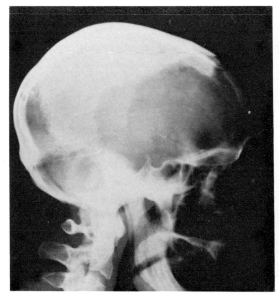

Plate 5.7

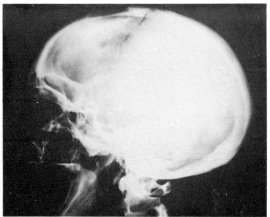

Plate 5.8

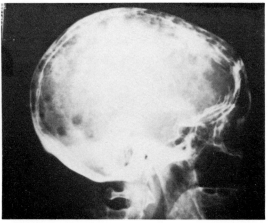

Plate 5.9

SOLUTIONS

Plate 5.1   Lateral view of adult skull following a road traffic accident. There is no evidence of fracture but there are several dense rectangular fragments over the upper part of the vault. These show the typical appearance of fragments of glass from a motor car windscreen and are embedded in either the scalp or the hair.

Plate 5.2   Lateral view of normal adult skull showing grooves for the middle meningeal artery on both sides, but not superimposed. Parieto-occipital sutures are visible, but the coronal suture is not well shown.

Plate 5.3   Baby's skull; note general under-development, unerupted teeth, and relatively wide, ill-defined sutures. An abnormal curvi-linear shadow, wider posteriorly, extends from the coronal suture to the back of the skull, and another, narrower, lower down, extends forwards a little way from the region of the lambda. This is an extensive fracture involving both parietal bones and encircling almost half the skull.

Plate 5.4   Normal adult skull (lateral view) showing venous channels in the diploë. Note edentulous upper jaw. Normal pituitary fossa is well shown, but the vault sutures are hardly visible.

Plate 5.5   Child's skull in lateral view (note un-erupted teeth and relatively underdeveloped facial bones) showing the so-called 'hair-on-end' appearance of numerous bone spicules protruding from the outer table of the frontal bone (and, to a lesser extent, from the back of the parietal bones). This is the typical appearance of the increased bone formation needed to support the additional bone marrow which develops in congenital haemolytic anaemia due to haemoglobinopathy, in this case homozygous SS disease. A similar picture is produced by other severe haemoglobinopathies such as thalassaemia major.

Plate 5.6   Adult skull, lateral view; there are numerous fillings in the upper teeth. There is irregular thickening of the inner table of the frontal bone the characteristic appearance of hyperostosis frontalis interna. The grooves for the middle meningeal artery and its branches are easily seen, and there are also similar grooves further back indicating a more posteriorly placed meningeal artery. The groove for the lateral sinus is also well seen, as are the soft-tissue shadows of the ears.

Plate 5.7   Adult skull, lateral view, edentulous. Much of the frontal, part of the parietal and part of the squamous occipital bones show marked thinning and increased transradiancy; the line of demarcation is relatively sharp. The intervening bone is normal. These appearances are characteristic of osteoporosis circumscripta of Paget's disease.

Plate 5.8   Adult skull, lateral view, edentulous. There is an expanding transradiant lesion in the vault of the skull in the region of the coronal suture. (A small dense opacity overlying the outer table further back is an extraneous object.) The lesion was due to a secondary deposit from carcinoma of the breast.

Plate 5.9   Adult skull, edentulous. The vault of the skull shows numerous rounded transradiancies of varying sizes having well-defined edges but no surrounding sclerotic rims and no expansion — the so-called 'punched-out' appearance. The vertical ramus of the mandible also shows an abnormal appearance with rather smaller transradiancies producing a generally irregular pattern. The appearances are typical of multiple myelomatosis.

BASE OF SKULL

The base of the skull should be traced systematically in the lateral view, starting at the anterior fossa and working backwards through the middle and posterior fossae.

Shape

In the lateral view note should be taken of the general shape of the base and, in particular, of two points of detail. The basal angle is formed between the floor of the anterior fossa and the back of the basisphenoid or clivus and should not normally exceed 140 degrees (the average has been given as 132 ± 4.6 degrees −1 standard

identify. Another method is that of Bull; lines drawn through the hard palate and the anterior and posterior arch of the atlas vertebra should be parallel in the normal. If there is much bone softening, in addition to platybasia there may be basilar invagination, in which the base of the skull appears to be draped over the cervical spine and the odontoid process is consequently well above its normal limits, and Bull's lines intersect, the hard palate rotating downwards (*Figure 5.3*).

Thickness

Increase in the thickness of any of the bones of the cranial fossae can occur in Paget's disease, fibrous dysplasia, basal meningioma (again, meningiomatous hyperostosis), neurofibromatosis, osteo-

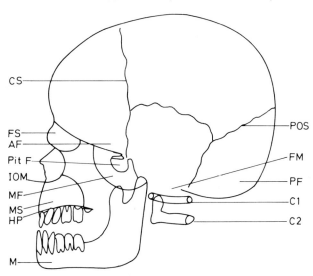

Figure 5.2   Diagram showing the principal radiological features in lateral view of the skull. Key as in Figure 5.1, plus:
AF–Anterior fossa
MF–Middle fossa
PF–Posterior fossa
Pit F–Pituitary fossa
HP–Hard palate

deviation). If this angle is increased the base is considered flattened and the term platybasia is appropriate. This is seen in a few congenital conditions such as mongolism and in conditions in which there is long-standing bone softening of the base, of which osteogenesis imperfecta, Paget's disease and osteomalacia are the classical examples. The other detail to note is the relationship of the odontoid process of the axis to the foramen magnum. There are several ways of assessing this but the simplest is to draw a line from the back of the hard palate to the posterior margin of the foramen magnum (Chamberlain's line); the odontoid process should not be more than 3 mm above this line. McGregor's line runs from the palate to the lowest point of the occiput, and is easier to

petrosis (in which the base is very dense and thick) and idiopathic hypercalcaemia (in which the base is not so thick and dense as in osteopetrosis but is relatively dense in comparison with the nearly normal vault − in the AP view the orbital margins are said to look like spectacles).

Decrease in thickness is seen generally in osteogenesis imperfecta, but local thinning is more common. There may be erosions of the middle fossa or of the basi-sphenoid by nasopharyngeal carcinoma, and of the clivus by the rare mid-line tumour chordoma. The middle fossa may be expanded and thinned by slow-growing cerebral tumour, possibly by aneurysm, or by a long-standing cystic lesion, of which one cause is a chronic subdural haematoma.

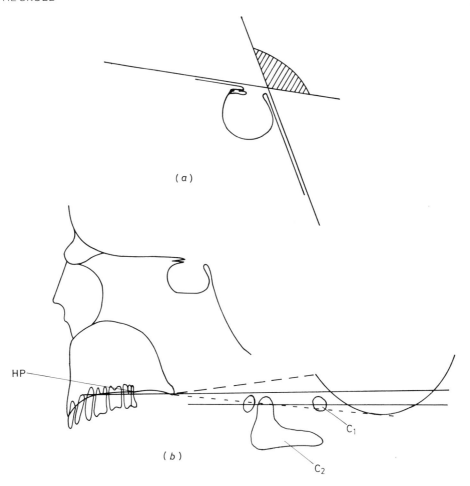

Figure 5.3 Diagrams showing some features of the base of the skull. (a) Basal angle, between the anterior fossa floor and the clivus or basisphenoid, which should not exceed 140 degrees. (b) Ways of showing basilar invagination.

– – – – – – *Chamberlain's line, from the back of the hard palate to the posterior rim of the foramen magnum; the odontoid process should not be more than 3 mm above it.*

- - - - - - - - - - *McGregor's line, from the back of the hard palate to the lowest point of the occipital bone.*

———————— *Bull's lines, through the hard palate and the anterior and posterior arch of the atlas, which should be parallel in the normal.*

Temporal bones

The temporal bones are shown in certain of the views in the sagittal plane, especially the straight PA view, the Towne's view and the submento-vertical or basal view. The internal auditory meati are well seen in the first two views; if there is an acoustic neuroma in the canal it may be widened or funnelled. Detail of the middle and inner ear is not easily seen on routine views and there are special views to show these, but they are very much the province of the radiologist and the otorhinolaryngologist. In the Towne's view, however, the mastoids are often well seen; clouding of the air cells is evidence of acute infection, and loss of the air cells with sclerosis indicates chronic infection. Destructive changes in the temporal bone may be due to extensive infection, sometimes accompanied by cholesteatoma (a relatively large transradiancy) or by local malignancy; two tumours may occur — carcinoma of middle ear or tumour of the glomus jugulare, but both are rare.

THE PITUITARY FOSSA (SELLA TURCICA)

This small but very important part of the skull should be looked at similarly in a systematic manner. It may be regarded in a lateral view as a rounded quadrilateral. The anterior wall and the floor are related to the sphenoid sinus and the posterior wall is the dorsum sellae. The posterior clinoid processes at the top of the dorsum sellae

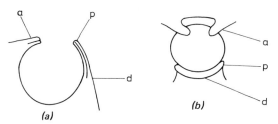

Figure 5.4 Diagrams showing the normal pituitary fossa (sella turcica); (a) in lateral view, (b) from above.
a. Anterior clinoid process
p. Posterior clinoid process
d. Dorsum sellae

are barely visible in a lateral view because they are directed laterally and only slightly forwards, but the anterior clinoic processes are well seen because they are directed backwards and medially; the interclinoid ligaments between them form the supports for the diaphragma sellae (which forms the roof) and may be calcified or even ossified (the so-called 'bridged sella'). The pituitary fossa should not exceed 14 mm in size in either height

or AP diameter, but it may be of more value to use the area calculated by multiplying these two figures. An area above 140 mm^2 may be regarded as suspicious and over 160 mm^2 as definitely abnormal. A small pituitary fossa is generally regarded as of no significance (see Figure 5.4). What matters most is the shape of the sella.

The fossa is difficult to see in views through the sagittal plane, but in Towne's view it is sometimes possible to see the dorsum sellae and the posterior clinoid processes through the foramen magnum, and in PA views the floor and the anterior clinoid processes can sometimes be made out through the ethmoid sinuses.

Systematic examination of the sella should start with a general look at the size and shape, any enlargement or variation being noted. The dorsum sellae should be examined for any change in angle or shape and for any loss of bone detail or actual defect or erosion. The floor and anterior wall should be checked for any evidence of expansion, ballooning or general enlargement of the sella and for loss of bone detail or erosion, and the anterior clinoid processes for evidence of erosion or even upward displacement.

There are two principal ways in which the sella becomes abnormal.

Rarefaction and/or erosion of the dorsum sellae
(Figure 5.5)

Raised intracranial tension has the effect of rendering the dorsum sellae rarefied, losing its fine

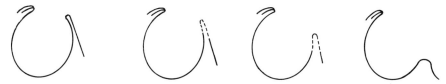

Figure 5.5 Diagrams showing the progressive rarefaction and erosion of the dorsum sellae, starting at the top, due to raised intracranial tension, culminating in its virtual disappearance.

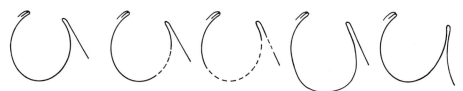

Figure 5.6 Diagrams showing the progressive erosion and enlargement of the floor of the pituitary end of the base of the dorsum sellae, the clinoid processes remaining intact, although sometimes they are displaced backwards.

cortical outlines. This usually starts from the top, and may progress until the whole of the posterior wall of the sellae has disappeared, but sometimes it is more uneven. Neighbouring tumours such as meningiomata, gliomata or metastatic or invasive carcinoma can also produce localized erosion. In all these situations the sella retains its general shape and the dorsum sellae is destroyed, in whole or in part, *in situ*.

Enlargement and/or change in shape of the sella (*Figure 5.6*)

Usually, as a result of an intrasellar tumour or cyst, commonly of the pituitary itself, the sella becomes expanded. The process starts by erosion of the floor and the adjacent part of the anterior or posterior wall, and continues to produce a ballooning of the border involved — forward or downward ballooning, or displacement backwards of the dorsum sellae. The dorsum sellae may, in part, become rarefied but it maintains its height. A craniopharyngioma may have the same effect because it may have an intrasellar element. A generalized enlargement of the sella may sometimes be seen in long-standing hydrocephalus, and other changes in shape may occur due to other adjacent tumours.

Calcification in the region of the sella is often helpful; in the interclinoid and petro-clinoid ligament it is normal, and a short linear shadow overlying the centre of the sella, due to an arteriosclerotic plaque in the carotid siphon, is common enough in older adults to be regarded as normal. Abnormal calcification above the sella is most commonly due to craniopharyngioma, but calcification above or round the sella may rarely be due to meningioma, glioma, aneurysm, angioma or possibly old tuberculous meningitis.

The interpretation of the more unusual variations in the shape of the pituitary fossa is very much a task for the specialist neuroradiologist, and the student should be well satisfied with recognizing a typical eroded dorsum sellae in raised intracranial tension, a typical ballooned sella of an intrasellar tumour, calcification associated with a craniopharyngioma, and the fact that other types of abnormalities exist which may need further investigation.

Some abnormalities of the base of the skull and/or the pituitary fossa are to be seen in *Plates 5.10–5.15*, but the other parts of the skull should also be inspected carefully.

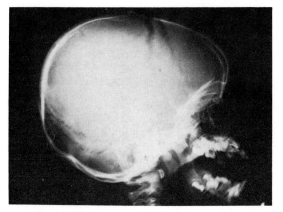

Plate 5.10

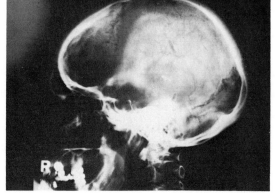
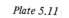

Plate 5.11

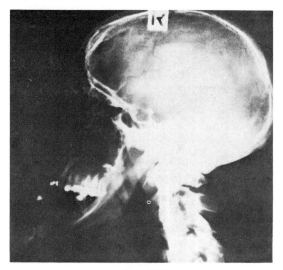

Plate 5.12

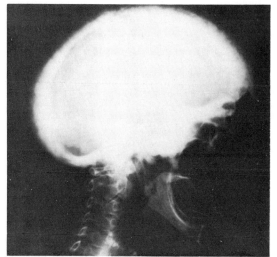

Plate 5.13

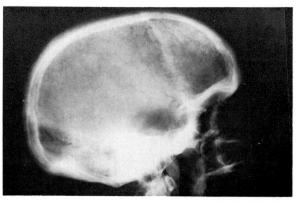

Plate 5.14

SOLUTIONS

Plate 5.10   Lateral view of a child's skull. Note the unerupted teeth and the underdeveloped facial bones. The pituitary fossa is difficult to see; the anterior clinoid processes are well shown, but the dorsum sellae is barely visible. There has been some rotation on the film so that this is not a true lateral view, as shown by the vertical rami of the mandible. The images of the coronal and parieto-occipital sutures on the two sides are separated; they show the increased width, blurring and zig-zag appearance typical of suture diastasis, and this, taken together with the disappearance of the dorsum sellae, indicates raised intracranial tension.

Plate 5.11   Lateral view of an adult skull. There are some fillings in the teeth. The pituitary fossa is enlarged, mostly in the antero-posterior direction. There is slight undercutting of the anterior wall beneath the anterior clinoid processes, and the dorsum sellae is thinner than usual and displaced backwards, the posterior clinoid processes being preserved. The posterior part of the floor also shows a double line, suggesting that it is displaced downwards asymmetrically. This film should be compared carefully with Plates 5.2, 5.4 and 5.6 which show absolutely normal pituitary fossae, and the differences will be evident. The lesion here is a pituitary tumour. The remainder of the skull is normal; venous markings in the vault and coronal and parieto-occipital sutures can be seen and the pineal is calcified; there are also some artefacts on the film.

Plate 5.12   Lateral view of an adult skull. Note that it is generally large. The pituitary fossa shows some general enlargement although its walls are intact without any erosion or rarefaction. The vault and base are normal but the frontal sinuses are large and prominent. The mandible is larger than usual with definite prognathus, that is, the lower incisor teeth (identified by an opaque filling) are in front of the upper. This is a typical appearance of acromegaly, but it is a case in which the pituitary fossa had received radiotherapy several years earlier, so that while the growth of the pituitary tumour had been arrested the increased size of the bones persisted.

Plate 5.13   Lateral view of an adult skull. There is gross 'woolly' thickening of the outer table of the vault with preservation of the normal inner table – typical of extensive Paget's disease. In addition, the base of the skull is also involved, is very dense and shows both platybasia and basilar invagination; the odontoid process is well above McGregor's line and just above Chamberlain's line, and Bull's lines are clearly not parallel. These observations can easily be checked with a transparent ruler, and compared with Figure 5.3.

Plate 5.14   Lateral view of an adult skull. The pituitary fossa is poorly defined and there is an erosion of the lower part of the dorsum sellae amounting to a definite defect, allowing the upper part to be displaced backwards. It is better seen on the enlargement in Plate 5.15. This is a good example of a relatively rapidly expanding intra-sellar pituitary tumour.

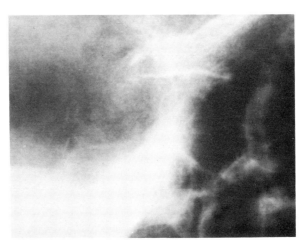

Plate 5.15

INTRACRANIAL CALCIFICATIONS

Normal

Calcification of the dura is very common and is of no significance; occasionally it is widespread, presenting a most confusing picture. More commonly it is confined to certain locations such as the interclinoid and petroclinoid ligaments, the edge of the tentorium, the dural walls of the sagittal sinus, and, commonest of all, the falx, visible in a PA view as a dense mid-line streak descending a few centimetres from the sagittal suture, but usually virtually invisible in a lateral view. The pineal is often calcified, and sometimes the habenular sommissure, just behind it, in the form of a 'C', open backwards; these should not be more than 3 mm from the mid-line. If displaced to one side (best shown on the Towne's view) a space-occupying lesion on the other side is almost always the cause. It should be noted that the falx is never displaced.

The choroid plexuses are sometimes calcified, lying above, lateral to and behind the pineal, and forming a triangle with it in a PA view. Each usually looks like a collection of dots, sometimes a well-defined oval, lying symmetrically, roughly in the middle of its half of the cerebrum.

Before trying to explain any intracranial calcification, then, it is important to check whether or not it lies in the position of any of the foregoing.

Abnormal

There are numerous causes of pathological intracranial calcification; unfortunately, in many of the cases the appearances are non-specific and diagnosis is difficult, but there are some pointers which may be of value. Many of the lesions are rare, and are very much the province of the specialist neuroradiologist.

A list of the causes of such lesions should at least include the following

Congenital: Tuberose sclerosis, lipoma of corpus callosum.

Traumatic: Old haematoma, subdural or extradural, recent or old foreign bodies (including scalp glass fragments).

Inflammatory: Toxoplasmosis, cytomegalic inclusion disease, sarcoidosis, tuberculosis.

Vascular: Aneurysm. vascular malformation, atheroma.

Neoplastic: Craniopharyngioma, glioma (astrocytoma, oligodendroglioma).

Metabolic: Hypoparathyroidism, pseudohypoparathyroidism (basal ganglia only).

The location of the lesion may assist in the diagnosis. Calcification in the region of the pituitary fossa has already been mentioned, and, if close to bone, old subdural haematoma or mengioma must be considered. The nature of the calcification may be more misleading than helpful. Curvilinear shadows may be seen symmetrically in the rare lipoma of the corpus callosum, and elsewhere in atheroma, haematoma and aneurysm. In infants and children, roughly symmetrical streaking or nodules would suggest toxoplasmosis or cytomegalic inclusion disease. In the Sturge—Weber syndrome (capillary naevus of meninges and of a corresponding skin area) curvilinear pairs of parallel lines are characteristic. Nodular shadowing may be seen in other lesions and amorphous masses of calcification may be due to inflammatory or neoplastic lesions. Hydatid cysts or cysticercosis nodules rarely calcify in the brain. It is important to exclude extraneous shadows (for example, in the scalp). Clearly, if an intracranial calcification does not fit easily into one of the known patterns, it requires further investigation to eliminate tumours, vascular lesions and infections. Unfortunately, most of these prove to be tumours.

Plates 5.16—5.20 show some examples of intracranial calcifications but also illustrate some other points of interest in the skull.

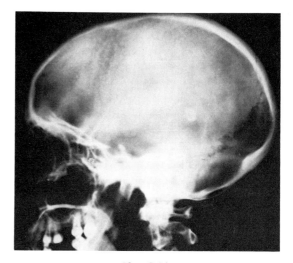

Plate 5.16

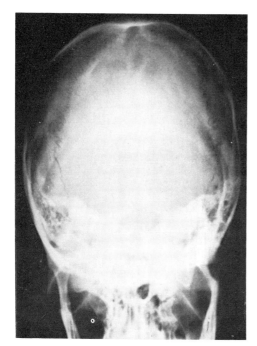

Plate 5.17

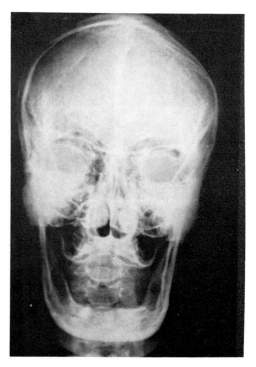

Plate 5.18

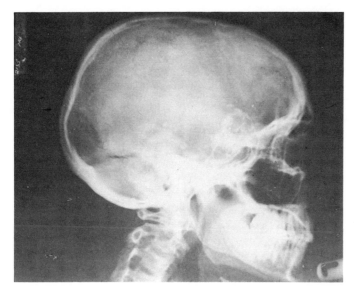

Plate 5.19

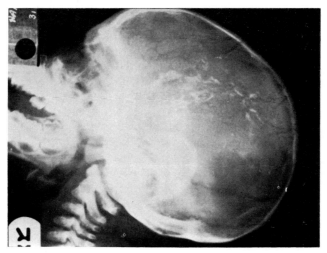

Plate 5.20

SOLUTIONS

Plate 5.16   Lateral view of normal adult skull. The vault shows the coronal and other sutures well with few vascular markings, and the rest of the skull, face and cervical spine look normal. The pineal is calcified, seen as a small dot above and behind the pituitary fossa, and above and behind this is an oval calcification, rather larger, one of the typical appearances of calcification in the choroid plexus. Since this is a good true lateral view, all the bilateral structures are accurately superimposed, and the two choroid plexuses thus produce a particularly dense shadow.

Plate 5.17   Same cases as in Plate 5.16, Towne's view. Coronal and parieto-occipital sutures are well seen, also the occipito-temporal sutures and the foramen magnum across the anterior part of which the top of the dorsum sellae is visible. In the squamous part of the occipital bone, the roughly cruciate shape of the torcula herophili or confluence of the sinuses can be made out, and superimposed on the lateral sinuses it is just possible to see the oval dense shadows of the calcified choroid plexuses. They appear less dense in this view than in the lateral view because each is seen separately. The film is slightly rotated, producing a slight apparent asymmetry, but the mandibular necks are well seen.

Plate 5.18   PA view of an edentulous adult skull with downward tilt of the x-ray beam. The petrous temporal bones still obscure the lower parts of the orbits and a little more tilt would have corrected this. The mandible is well seen but the necks are obscured in this view. The vault of the skull is relatively featureless but a dense shadow in the upper part of the cranial cavity is due to calcification of the falx cerebri.

Plate 5.19   Lateral view of an adult skull. The vault shows normal sutures and venous markings but there is extensive irregular calcification above and slightly in front of the pituitary fossa which is slightly ballooned with a thinned dorsum sellae. The pineal is calcified and in normal position. The rest of the skull is normal with normal dentition. Appearances are typical of craniopharyngioma.

Plate 5.20   Lateral view of a child's skull with some rotation, as shown by the separation of the mandibular necks and of the parieto-occipital sutures on the two sides and also of the ears. Numerous unerupted teeth. Scattered irregular calcification within the cranial cavity was in this case due to toxoplasmosis (as shown by the complement fixation reaction), but the appearances would do equally well for cytomegalic inclusion disease.

FACIAL REGION

Here the radiological anatomy is somewhat complicated since the various structures overlap in the various views, so that detailed interpretation is frequently the province of the radiologist and the oral or otorhinolaryngological surgeon. However, some basic observations may be made without a too deep involvement in detail.

A lateral view does not present too much difficulty provided it is examined systematically in the following sequence; frontal sinuses, nasal bones, ethmoid sinuses, sphenoid sinus, maxillary sinuses, hard palate, teeth and tongue, pharyngeal airway and mandible. The views through the sagittal plane are of more value but are more difficult. For the sinuses an occipito-mental (OM) view (a PA view with the head tilted upwards at an angle of about 45 degrees) is usually enough and the frontal sinuses and antra are well shown. In traumatic cases it is usual to tilt the tube 30 degrees downwards and take a second film which shows the inferior orbital margin and the antral walls rather better. For the mandible, a PA view and both oblique views are usually taken which display the anatomy satisfactorily. In addition, a Towne's view centred rather lower than usual is very valuable in showing the zygomatic arches and the necks and condyles of the mandible.

Sinuses

If any of the sinuses become filled with fluid they become relatively opaque in comparison with the rest of the face since they acquire radiographic water density; the fluid may, of course, be clear fluid, pus or blood. An air—fluid level is sometimes seen. If the mucosal lining is thickened, then it shows as a lesser density (not so thick as the whole depth of the sinus), but it is still more dense than the remaining air which can be seen as a transradiancy in the centre of the sinus. Sometimes the mucosa is thickened in one place only when it tends to form a round mass attached to one wall, a polyp, usually associated with allergic conditions. If the sinus is opaque and there is erosion of one of its walls, then malignant disease may be suspected. The antrum may also fill with blood if one of its walls are fractured — a common association. An ivory osteoma sometimes occurs in a frontal sinus.

Upper facial bones

Congenital, inflammatory, vascular and neoplastic lesions of the face usually present clinically; they rapidly become the province of the oral or otorhinolaryngological surgeon and subject to specialist radiology. It is, however, important for the student to become familiar with the appearances of the common fracture of the facial bones, since after injury soft-tissue swelling may rapidly conceal the true nature of the damage which can only be shown radiologically. These should not be missed; delay in treatment may result in permanent deformity and/or disability.

Fractures of the nasal bones are made more difficult to diagnose by the presence normally of relatively deep grooves (usually two oblique and one short horizontal) which are vascular and should not be mistaken for fractures. True fractures will cross these grooves and there should be some displacement. If lateral, this should be visible on the OM film.

The full classification of types of facial fracture, which are the province of the maxillo-facial surgeon and the radiologist, is out of place here, but essentially there are lateral and central fractures. The common lateral fracture is the depressed fracture of the zygomatic malar bone which has some characteristic features. The fronto-malar synchondrosis is opened out, there is a step in the inferior orbital margin, there is a fracture of the lateral wall of the antrum and a fracture of the zygomatic arch, and frequently the antrum is opaque due to blood. It usually requires a combination of OM, tilted OM and Towne's views to demonstrate the full picture.

In the lateral view of central fractures there is some degree of backward displacement and tilting of the antrum, the palate and the teeth-bearing alveolus, and in the views through the sagittal plane there is always some damage to the orbits or antra, or both.

Mandible

Mandibular fractures may occur in the neck, at the angle or through the mental foramen. Very frequently there are two fractures since the bone forms a ring with the skull, say, mental foramen and neck. The key to recognizing fractures of the neck is to check the angle it makes with the skull in the PA and Towne's views. It should be roughly perpendicular.

Airway

Lateral views of the skull also show the dark shadow of the air-filled pharynx. Although special lateral views of this region are needed for good detail, for example, to show the larynx and surrounding structures and the tonsils and adenoids in children, some information is available on a skull film.

THE CERVICAL SPINE

The cervical spine is not particularly well shown on standard views of the skull, and may present a confusing appearance unless specifically noted. In a lateral view of the skull the atlas vertebra is seen in lateral view, but it is usually rotated on the axis vertebra, which is consequently seen in oblique view. There is some degree of obliquity of the rest of the cervical vertebrae. The relationships of the upper articular facets of the atlas vertebra to the occipital condyles should be noted (subluxation can occur) and also the relationship of the odontoid process of the axis to the anterior arch of the atlas. If the ligaments keeping these two bones in contact are damaged by trauma or weakened by disease (for example, rheumatoid disease and occasionally severe tonsillitis in children) the resulting atlanto-axial subluxation or dislocation can produce spinal cord damage or even transection from backward pressure of the odontoid.

It is sometimes possible to see obvious abnormalities such as gross injuries or defects, or extensive osteoarthritic changes. In the PA views, the lower cervical spine is adequately shown, though it may be rather dark on account of the greater exposure required for the skull. The odontoid process is often seen through the foramen magnum, with the anterior arch of the atlas in front of it, on the OM and submento-vertical (SMV or basal) views, and the posterior arch of the atlas in the Towne's view.

It is particularly important to inspect the cervical vertebrae in cases of head injury and if vertebral bony damage is suspected there are good grounds for requesting formal views of the cervical spine.

Plates 5.21—5.23 show some facial appearances of interest.

167

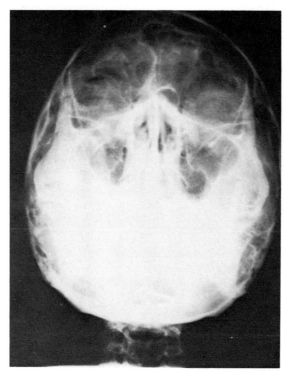

Plate 5.21

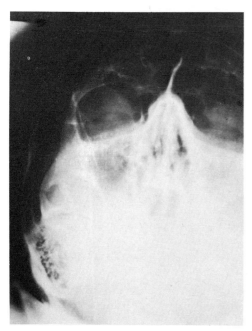

Plate 5.22

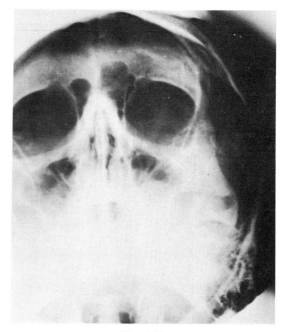

Plate 5.23

SOLUTIONS

Plate 5.21   Adult skull; occipito-mental view to show the facial bones. The left side is normal but on the right the fronto-malar synchondrosis has opened, as shown by a narrow transradiancy which has appeared. There is a step in the inferior orbital margin and increased dense shadowing in the region of the cheek. The zygomatic or malar bone is depressed, as can be shown by placing a ruler horizontally across the film, and it is just possible to see that the lateral wall of the antrum is fractured. The antrum still contains air but there is a shadow in its lateral part, probably due to a submucosal haematoma.

Plate 5.22   Normal skull; occipito-mental view to show the sinuses. The frontal sinuses are extensive but normal, as is the right antrum, but the left antrum shows general thickening of its lining membrane, otherwise known as mucosal thickening, and usually due to infection.

Plate 5.23   Normal skull; occipito-mental view to show the sinuses. The frontal sinuses are small but normal and the right antrum is normal. The left antrum shows a rounded shadow arising from its floor. This is due to localized or polypoid thickening of the mucosa, more commonly associated with allergic conditions. The appearances of the left antrum in this and Plate 5.22 should be compared and contrasted.

Bibliography

Suggested books for further reading

The list of books which follows is not intended to be exhaustive, but it includes a number of standard works in the English language which are likely to be found in a hospital or university library. The larger ones are clearly unsuitable for systematic study by an undergraduate, or even a clinical postgraduate student, although they fall into the province of the trainee radiologist. A short observation alongside each is not intended to be a formal criticism of the work, but to show how it might benefit the student, based to some extent on the great value they have been (albeit in earlier editions!) to the writer of the present work.

GENERAL RADIOLOGY

Kreel, L. (1971). *An Outline of Radiology* (concise and containing much material; no x-rays reproduced but many helpful diagrams)

Sante, L. R. (1956). *Principles of Roentgenologic Interpretation* (Out of print). Michigan; Edwards Brothers Inc. (Readable and easy to refer to; contains many diagrams and valuable sections on heart disease and bone lesions)

Shanks, S. C. and Kerley, P. (Eds) *A Text-book of X-ray Diagnosis by British Authors,* 4th ed. London; Lewis. In six volumes: I. *The Head and Neck* (1969); II. *The Cardiovascular System* (1972); III. *The Respiratory System* (1973); IV. *The Alimentary Tract* (1969); V. *The Abdomen* (1970); and VI. *Bones, Joints and Soft Tissues* (1971) (the standard work in British radiology; extensive, and unlikely to have any significant omissions)

Simon, G. (1975). *X-Ray Diagnosis for Clinical Students and Practitioners,* 3rd ed. London; Butterworths (an introduction to radiology, with more about the x-ray department)

Squire, Lucy F. (1964). *Fundamentals of Roentgenology.* Cambridge, Mass; Harvard University Press

Sutton, D. (1976). *Radiology for General Practitioners and Medical Students,* 3rd ed. London; Churchill-Livingstone (a small book in paperback form giving a wide-ranging introduction to radiology)
and Grainger, R. G. (1974). *Text book of Radiology,* 2nd ed. London; Churchill-Livingstone (a complete textbook of radiology in one volume. Concise and to the point)

Troupin, Rosalind H. (1974). *Diagnostic Radiology in Clinical Medicine.* London; Lloyd-Luke (a short book containing a lot of useful material)

CHEST

Simon, G. (1978). *Principles of Chest X-Ray Diagnosis,* 4th ed. London; Butterworths (based on radiological appearances rather than anatomy or aetiology – a standard work)

ABDOMEN

Frijmann Dahl, L. (1974). *Roentgen Examination in Acute Abdominal Disease,* 3rd ed. (the major work on this subject)

Gough, M. H., and Gear, M. W. L. (1971). *The Plain X-Ray in the Diagnosis of the Acute Abdomen.* Oxford; Blackwell (a surgical handbook with notes on clinical presentation and differential diagnosis)

Ryan, M. J. (1969). *Moments with Diagnostic Radiology,* Vol. 1: *The Abdomen.* London, New York and Toronto; Saunders (a small paperback book with excellent radiographs reproduced as problems with pertinent commentaries)

BONES

Edeiken and Hodes (1974). *Roentgen Diagnosis of Diseases of Bones* (in 2 Vols.). Baltimore; Williams and Wilkins (the original book, being the 'bones' section (by Pugh) of a larger work edited by Ross Goolden, is a full but relatively succinct account of radiology of bone disease. The later work, with two editors, is more extensive and complete, in two volumes)

Jacobs, P. (1973). *Atlas of Hand Radiographs.* London; Harvey, Miller and Metcalf (beautifully illustrated to show local and general disease manifested in the hand)

Pugh, D. (1951). *Roentgenologic Diagnosis of Diseases of Bones.* Baltimore; Williams and Wilkins (*see* Edeiken and Hodes)

Simon, G. (1973). *Principles of Bone X-Ray Diagnosis,* 3rd ed. London; Butterworths (based on radiological appearances rather than anatomy or aetiology)

SKULL

du Boulay, G. H. (1965). *Principles of X-Ray Diagnosis of the Skull.* London; Butterworths (extensive consideration of skull radiology, based on radiological appearances − 2nd edition in preparation)

PAEDIATRICS

Caffey, J. (1972). *Pediatric X-Ray Diagnosis,* 6th ed., in 2 Vols. Chicago; Year Book Publishers (the standard major work on the subject)

TROPICAL DISEASES

Middlemiss, H. (Ed.) (1961). *Tropical Radiology.* London; Heinemann (chapters on special subjects, including tropical parasites)

Index